CONTENTS

Copyright

Introduction

Section I Understanding Cancer   1

Chapter 1 The Eight Hallmarks of Cancer   2

Chapter 2 How does the Human Body Fight Against Cancer   10

Chapter 3 When Cancer Become Deadly: Benign vs Malignant Tumors   27

Section II Understanding Six Major Options for Cancer Treatment   35

Chapter 4 Surgery as a Cancer Treatment Option   38

Chapter 5 Radiation Therapy as a Cancer Treatment Option   52

Chapter 6 Chemotherapy as a Cancer Treatment Option   58

Chapter 7 Targeted Therapy as a Cancer Treatment Option   70

Chapter 8 Immunotherapy as a Cancer Treatment Option   79

Chapter 9 Integrative and Alternative Treatment on Cancer as an Option   90

Chapter 10 Frontiers of Cancer Treatment Development   95

Section III Cancer Patient Nutrition, Diet and Off-Label Drug Use   102

Chapter 11 Key Nutrients and Nutrition Strategies for   104

Cancer Patients

Chapter 12   Anti-inflammatory Diet, DASH Diet,   116
Mediterranean Diet and Vegetarian Diet

Chapter 13   Nutrition that can boost one's immune   131
system

Chapter 14 Off-label Drug Use for Cancer Treatment   146

Section IV   Selecting the Cancer Treatment Team and   151
Treatment Center

Chapter 15 Key Considerations when Selecting Cancer   153
Treatment Team and Facility

Chapter 16 Top-Ranked US Cancer Treatment Centers   187

Section V Managing Cancer Treatment Costs   200

Chapter 17   Cancer Care with Private Insurance,   203
Obamacare and Medicare

Chapter 18 Strategies to Save Money on Cancer Care   208

Section VI   Supporting Cancer Patients and Survivors   215
with Palliative Care

Chapter 19 Understanding Palliative Care   218

Chapter 20 Catering Palliative Care to a Specific Cancer   224
Treatment Provided

Chapter 21 Hospice Care   237

Section VII   Creating an Action Plan after Cancer   240
Diagnosis

Chapter 22   Understand the Diagnosis and Choose a   243
Trusted Treatment Team

Chapter 23 Build a Solid Support Network and Prepare for   256
Treatment

Chapter 24 Create a Backup Plan and Communicate with   266
Loved Ones

About The Author   275

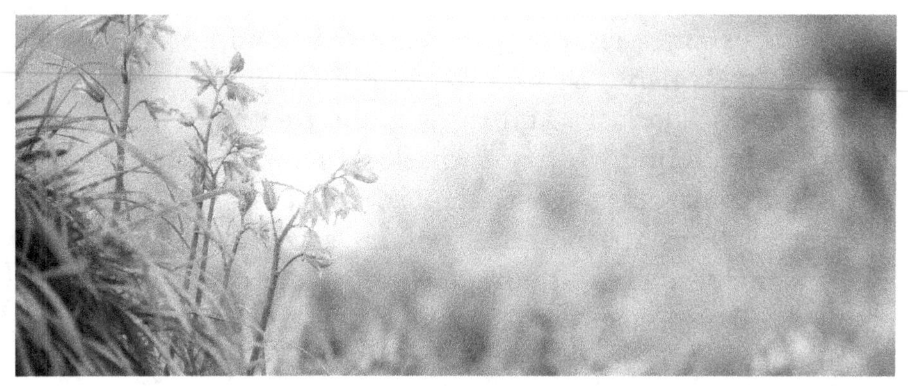

INTRODUCTION

Cancer is a global health challenge that affects millions of people around the world. It is a disease that knows no boundaries, affecting individuals regardless of age, gender, race, or socioeconomic status. Nearly 9 million people a year lose their lives to cancer in the world. In the US, it is the second most common cause of death.

In the face of a cancer diagnosis, navigating the complex landscape of treatment options can be overwhelming and bewildering. Fortunately, over the years, the field of oncology has made tremendous strides in understanding the biology of cancer and developing innovative therapies. This book is designed to provide you with a comprehensive understanding of modern cancer treatments, empowering you to make informed decisions and take an active role in your own care or that of a loved one.

In this book, we will explore a wide range of topics, from the fundamentals of cancer biology to the cutting-edge technologies and therapies that are transforming the way we approach treatment. We will delve into the different types of cancer, their diagnosis, and the various treatment modalities available, including surgery, radiation therapy, chemotherapy, immunotherapy, targeted therapies, and precision medicine. The book places special emphasis on several most common cancers, including breast, lung, prostate, colorectal, pancreatic, etc. We will also discuss the important role of supportive care, the integration of complementary and alternative therapies, and the impact of lifestyle choices on cancer prevention and survivorship.

The aim of this book is not only to educate, but also to provide practical advice and guidance to patients, their families, and caregivers. Cancer treatment involves a multidisciplinary approach, and we delve into the roles of various healthcare professionals, such as oncologists, surgeons, radiologists, nurses, and psychologists, who work together as a team to provide personalized care.

Throughout the book, we emphasize the importance of shared decision-making and patient-centered care. We understand that every person's journey with cancer is unique, and there is no one-size-fits-all approach. By equipping you with knowledge about the available options, potential side effects, and strategies for managing treatment-related challenges, we aim to empower you to actively participate in your treatment plan.

We recognize that this book cannot replace the individualized guidance and care provided by your cancer treatment team. Instead, it serves as a companion to your journey, offering you a comprehensive understanding of modern cancer treatments and serving as a reference to help you engage in meaningful discussions with your healthcare providers.

We hope that this book will serve as a valuable resource,

instilling confidence, providing clarity, and offering support during a challenging time. By combining scientific knowledge with practical advice, we aim to empower you to make informed decisions and optimize the outcomes of your cancer treatment. Remember, you are not alone on this journey, and together, we can navigate the path toward hope, healing, and a better future.

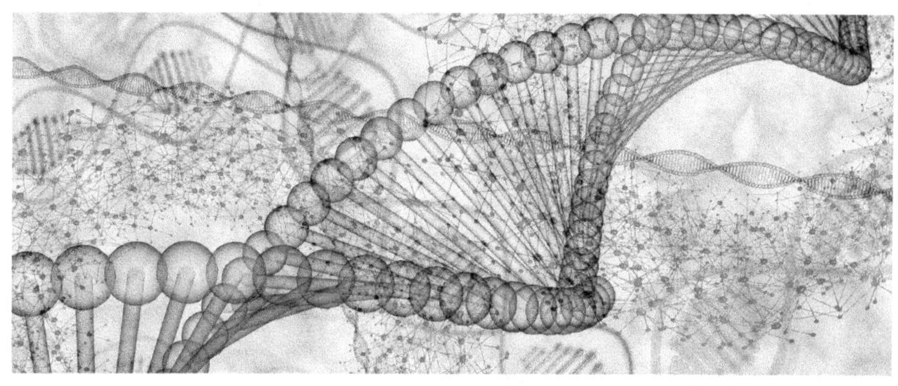

SECTION I UNDERSTANDING CANCER

ancer is a disease that has been affecting humans for centuries. Cancer is a heavy topic that evokes both misconceptions and fear due to its devastating impact on individuals and society as a whole. Misconceptions arise from a lack of understanding and inaccurate information, leading to myths and misconceptions about the causes, treatment options, and outcomes of cancer. These misconceptions can fuel fear and anxiety, as people may believe that cancer is always a death sentence or that there are no effective treatments available. Additionally, the fear of cancer stems from its unpredictable nature and the potential for significant physical, emotional, and financial burdens. The fear of losing loved ones, the uncertainty of one's own health, and the potential for painful treatments and side effects contribute to the heaviness associated with cancer, making it a topic that demands accurate information, empathy, and support.

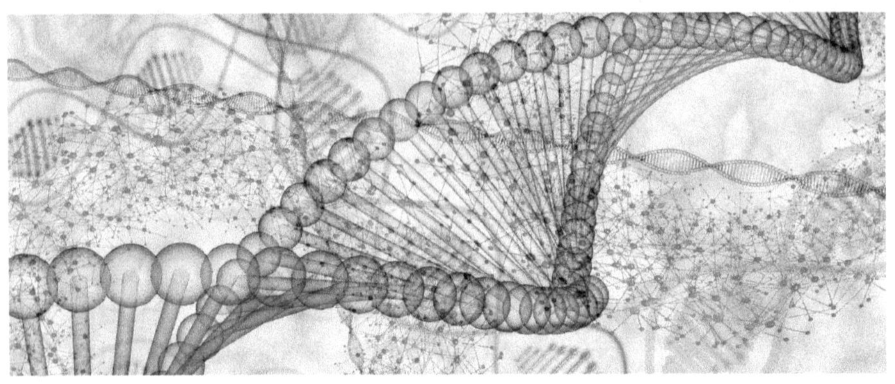

CHAPTER 1 THE EIGHT HALLMARKS OF CANCER

Cancer is a complex and multifaceted disease that affects millions of people worldwide. Despite advances in medicine and technology, cancer continues to be a leading cause of death, making it an important area of research for scientists and healthcare professionals. In this chapter, we will explore the eight known hallmarks of cancer, the progress on cancer research and the latest understanding of cancer on both molecular and cellular levels.

The Eight Hallmarks of Cancer

In 2000, Douglas Hanahan and Robert Weinberg proposed the "Hallmarks of Cancer" hypothesis, which outlined the fundamental characteristics of cancer cells. They identified six hallmarks that cancer cells must possess to develop into a tumor: sustained proliferation, evasion of growth suppressors, resistance to cell death, replicative immortality, induction of angiogenesis, and invasion and metastasis. In 2011, they added two additional hallmarks: deregulating cellular energetics and evading the immune system.

1. Sustained Proliferation: Normal cells have a finite lifespan and divide only when necessary. Cancer cells, on the other hand, divide uncontrollably, resulting in the formation of a tumor.

2. Evasion of Growth Suppressors: Normal cells are regulated by growth suppressor genes that prevent them from dividing when they shouldn't. Cancer cells often have mutations in these genes, allowing them to bypass these checkpoints and continue to divide.

3. Resistance to Cell Death: Normal cells undergo programmed cell death (apoptosis) when they are damaged or no longer needed. Cancer cells can resist apoptosis, allowing them to continue to grow and divide.

4. Replicative Immortality: Normal cells have a limited lifespan and can only divide a certain number of times before dying. Cancer cells, however, can continue to divide indefinitely, giving rise to an immortal cell line.

5. Induction of Angiogenesis: Tumors need a blood supply to grow, and cancer cells can induce the formation of new blood vessels to support their growth.

6. Invasion and Metastasis: Cancer cells can break away from the primary tumor and invade surrounding tissues, as well as spread to other parts of the body through the bloodstream or lymphatic system.

7. Deregulating Cellular Energetics: Cancer cells can alter their metabolism to support their rapid growth and division.

8. Evading the Immune System: Cancer cells can evade the immune system, allowing them to continue to grow and spread without being detected.

Progress on Cancer Research

Over the years, significant progress has been made in the field of cancer research. This progress has been driven by a number of factors, including: 1) The development of new technologies, such as next-generation sequencing, which has allowed researchers to better understand the genetic basis of cancer and facilitate diagnosis of cancer biomarkers; 2) The development of new drugs and treatments, such as targeted therapies and immunotherapy, which have improved the survival rates for many types of cancer; 3) The development of new clinical trials, which have allowed researchers to test new treatments and identify the best treatments for each type of cancer.

We now know that cancer is caused by a combination of genetic and environmental factors, and that it can arise from mutations in oncogenes (genes that promote cell growth) or tumor suppressor genes (genes that prevent cell growth). In fact, researchers have identified many oncogenes and tumor suppressor genes that play a role in the development and progression of cancer. Cancer is a disease of the genome with numerous mutations in the DNA of cells, with specific mutations in cancer cells driving the development and progression of certain types of cancer.

In addition, researchers have discovered that cancer is not a single disease, but rather a collection of diseases that can be classified based on the affected tissue type and the specific genetic mutations that are driving the cancer. On a cellular level, cancer cells have altered signaling pathways that allow them to bypass the normal checkpoints that regulate cell growth and division. They also have changes in their metabolism that allow them to use glucose and other nutrients more efficiently, providing them with the energy they need. In addition, studies have shown that the tumor microenvironment, which includes the surrounding blood vessels, immune cells, and extracellular matrix, plays a critical role in the development and progression of cancer. Understanding these mechanisms is crucial for developing new therapies and improving patient outcomes.

In the realm of lung cancer, researchers have made

noteworthy progress in identifying specific genetic mutations and biomarkers associated with the disease. This has led to the development of targeted therapies, such as tyrosine kinase inhibitors, which have shown remarkable effectiveness in certain subsets of patients. Immunotherapy has also emerged as a promising treatment avenue, with immune checkpoint inhibitors demonstrating improved outcomes in advanced lung cancer patients. For example, the drug pembrolizumab (Keytruda) has been shown to improve survival rates for patients with advanced lung cancer who have no other treatment options.

Breast cancer research has witnessed significant advancements in personalized medicine. The development of new screening methods, such as mammograms, has led to earlier detection of breast cancer, which has improved survival rates. Scientists are also leveraging genomic profiling techniques to identify the unique genetic characteristics of individual tumors. This allows for more tailored treatment approaches, including targeted therapies and hormone receptor-based therapies. Furthermore, novel immunotherapeutic strategies, such as immune-modulating drugs and vaccines, are being explored to enhance the body's immune response against breast cancer cells.

In the case of colon cancer, research efforts are focused on early detection and prevention. Screening methods like colonoscopy, stool-based cancer biomarker detection and genetic testing have played a crucial role in identifying individuals at high risk. Additionally, advancements in understanding the genetic and molecular mechanisms of colon cancer have led to the development of targeted therapies and immunotherapies. Combination therapies, including chemotherapy and immunotherapy, are being investigated to improve treatment outcomes.

Prostate cancer research has seen notable progress in precision medicine approaches. Newer diagnostic techniques, such as multiparametric MRI, prostate-specific antigen (PSA) tests and liquid biopsies, are improving the accuracy of prostate cancer detection and monitoring. Targeted therapies, such as androgen receptor pathway inhibitors, are being utilized to block specific molecular pathways involved in prostate cancer growth. Immunotherapies, including cancer vaccines and immune checkpoint inhibitors, are also under investigation to bolster the immune response against prostate cancer cells.

Pancreatic cancer remains one of the most challenging forms of cancer to treat. However, researchers are focusing on developing more effective diagnostic tools, including liquid biopsies and imaging techniques, to detect pancreatic cancer at earlier stages. Novel treatment strategies, such as targeted therapies, immunotherapies, and combination approaches, are being explored to improve survival rates and enhance patient outcomes. For example, the drug gemcitabine (Gemzar) has been shown to improve survival rates for patients with pancreatic cancer.

Overall, cancer research has made significant progress in understanding the molecular basis of different types of cancer and developing targeted therapies. As a result of this progress, the overall cancer death rate in the United States has declined by 25% since 1991. Ongoing efforts continue to push the boundaries of knowledge, with the ultimate goal of improving prevention, early detection, and treatment options for patients across the spectrum of cancer types.

Cancer Risk Factors

Researchers have also found that there are many contributing factors that can increase the risk of cancer development, with most common risk factors including genetic susceptibility, environmental factors, age, diet choice and underlying medical conditions.

1) Genetic Susceptibility and Cancer

One of the most significant risk factors for developing cancer is a genetic predisposition. This means that individuals with certain genes have a higher likelihood of developing cancer than those without these genes. Some of the most well-known cancer susceptibility genes are BRCA1 and BRCA2, which are associated with a higher risk of breast and ovarian cancer.

Other cancer susceptibility genes include TP53, which is associated with a higher risk of several types of cancer, including breast, ovarian, and colorectal cancer, and APC, which is associated with a higher risk of colorectal cancer. In addition to these well-known cancer susceptibility genes, there are many other genes that can increase an individual's risk of developing cancer.

Other genetic conditions, such as Lynch syndrome and familial adenomatous polyposis, can increase the risk of colorectal and other cancers.

It is essential to understand one's family history of cancer and whether they have a predisposition to certain types of cancer. Genetic testing is available for some genetic mutations, allowing individuals to understand their risk and take preventive measures to reduce their cancer risk. Also, while having a genetic predisposition to cancer can increase an individual's risk, it does not necessarily mean that they will develop the disease. Other factors, such as environmental factors and lifestyle choices, also play a significant role in cancer development.

2) Environmental Factors and Cancer

Environmental factors are another major risk factor for cancer development. These factors include exposure to chemicals, radiation, and other harmful substances. Exposure to toxins, radiation, and pollution can damage cells, leading to cancer growth. One of the most well-known environmental factors associated with cancer is cigarette smoking, which is responsible for significant lung cancer cases as well as for an estimated 30% of all cancer deaths.

Other environmental factors that can increase an individual's risk of cancer include exposure to chemicals such as benzene and asbestos, as well as radiation exposure, such as from X-rays. For example, exposure to UV radiation from the sun or tanning beds can increase the risk of skin cancer.

In addition to these factors, pollution and poor air quality have also been linked to an increased risk of cancer. These environmental factors can cause changes in the body's cells, which can lead to cancer development over time.

3) Age and Cancer

Age is another significant risk factor for cancer development. As we age, our cells are more likely to accumulate genetic mutations, which can increase the risk of cancer development. In addition, the body's immune system may become less effective at identifying and eliminating cancer cells as we age, further increasing the risk of cancer.

Some types of cancer, such as prostate and breast cancer, are more common in older individuals. It is important for individuals of all ages to be aware of their risk for cancer and to take steps to reduce their risk, such as getting regular cancer screenings and maintaining a healthy lifestyle. Regular screenings can be critical in identifying cancer early, especially for individuals over the age of 50. Mammograms, colonoscopies, and other cancer screenings can detect cancer in its early stages, allowing for prompt treatment and improved outcomes.

4) Diet Choice and Cancer

Diet choice can also play a role in cancer development. Eating a diet high in red and processed meats has been linked to an increased risk of colorectal cancer. In contrast, a diet rich in fruits, vegetables, and whole grains have been shown to reduce the risk of several types of cancer, including breast, lung, and colorectal cancer. Alcohol consumption, especially in excess, can increase the risk of liver, breast, and other cancers.

In addition, maintaining a healthy weight and engaging in regular physical activity can also help reduce the risk of cancer. Obesity has been linked to an increased risk of several types of cancer, including breast, colorectal, and kidney cancer, as excess body fat can produce hormones that can promote cancer growth.

5) Medical Conditions

Underlying medical conditions can also increase the risk of cancer development. For example, individuals with chronic hepatitis B or C infections are at a higher risk of developing liver cancer. Additionally, individuals with ulcerative colitis or Crohn's disease are at an increased risk of developing colorectal cancer.

Overall, there are many factors that can increase an individual's risk of cancer, including genetic predisposition, environmental factors, age, and diet choice. While cancer risk factors are complex and multifactorial, understanding them can help individuals take preventive measures to reduce their risk. Genetic testing, lifestyle changes, regular screenings, and healthy dietary choices can all play a role in reducing one's risk of cancer development. By taking proactive steps to reduce their risk, individuals can improve their overall health and potentially avoid cancer altogether.

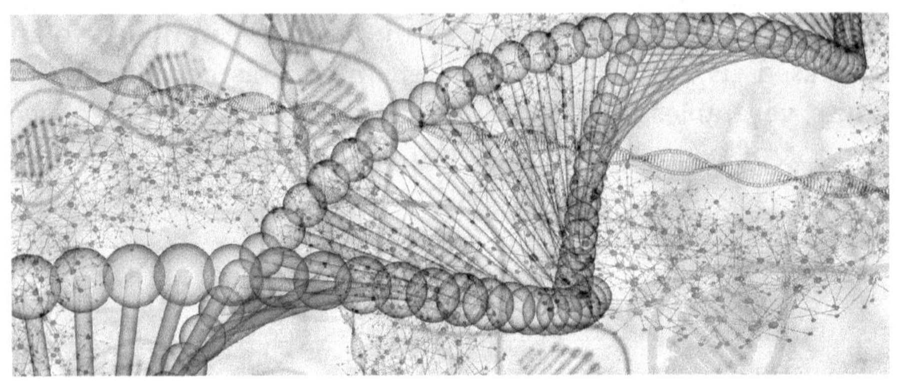

CHAPTER 2 HOW DOES THE HUMAN BODY FIGHT AGAINST CANCER

Although cancer is a disease in which cells grow abnormally and spread rapidly to other parts of the body, the human body has a number of natural defenses against cancer. These defenses include:

- The immune system network: The immune system network is a complex network of cells, tissues, and organs that work together to protect the body from infection. The immune system can also recognize and destroy cancer cells.

- The DNA repair system: The DNA repair system is responsible for repairing damaged DNA. When DNA is damaged, it can lead to cancer. The DNA repair system helps to prevent this by repairing damaged DNA before it can cause cancer.

- Apoptosis: Apoptosis is a natural process of cell death.

When cells die by apoptosis, they are broken down and recycled by the body. Cancer cells can also undergo apoptosis. However, cancer cells often have defects in their apoptosis pathways, which allows them to survive and grow.

Typically, when the natural defenses are having an upper hand against cancer cells, cancer cells are eliminated; however, when these natural defenses are not strong enough due to a variety of factors including the risk factors discussed in previous chapter, cancer cells, through accumulated mutations over many years, can evade the immune system, damage the DNA repair system, or prevent apoptosis. When this happens, cancer can continue to grow unchecked.

The Immune System Network as a Natural Defense against Cancer

The immune system, which is made up of various organs, cells, and molecules, is one of the natural defenses responsible for identifying and destroying cancer cells before they have a chance to grow and spread. Individuals with a strong immune system is usually better equipped to fight off cancer cells. Additionally, some individuals may have genetic variations that provide increased protection against cancer or help the immune system identify and destroy cancer cells more effectively.

In this complex network of cells, tissues, and organs of the immune system, the key components are white blood cells (leukocytes), antibodies, and other molecules that work together to identify and destroy cancer cells.

One of the primary organs in the immune system is the bone marrow, which is responsible for producing various types of white blood cells. White blood cells are the key players in the immune system and are responsible for recognizing and destroying cancer cells. There are several types of white blood cells, including T-cells, B-cells, natural killer cells, and macrophages. Each type of white blood cell has a specific function in the immune system's defense against cancer.

T-cells are a type of white blood cell that is responsible for recognizing and destroying cancer cells. They identify cancer cells by recognizing specific proteins on their surface called antigens. Once the T-cells identify a cancer cell, they release chemicals called cytokines that signal other immune cells to attack the cancer cell. B-cells are another type of white blood cell that produces antibodies, which are proteins that can identify and neutralize cancer cells.

Natural killer cells are a type of white blood cell that can recognize and destroy cancer cells without the need for specific antigen recognition. They are called "natural killers" because they can recognize and kill cancer cells on their own. Macrophages are another type of white blood cell that can engulf and destroy cancer cells. They also produce cytokines that activate other immune cells to attack cancer cells.

In lung cancer, immune cells such as T cells, natural killer (NK) cells, and dendritic cells are central to the immune response. T cells, specifically cytotoxic T lymphocytes (CTLs), recognize and eliminate cancer cells by recognizing tumor-specific antigens presented on the surface of cancer cells. NK cells are responsible for directly killing cancer cells and releasing cytokines that enhance the immune response. Dendritic cells capture and process antigens from cancer cells, presenting them to T cells to activate an immune response. Immune checkpoint molecules, such as PD-1 and CTLA-4, also play a role in lung cancer by regulating the T cell response, and immune checkpoint inhibitors have shown efficacy in restoring anti-tumor immunity.

In breast cancer, immune cells within the tumor microenvironment, including T cells, B cells, and macrophages, contribute to the immune response. Tumor-infiltrating lymphocytes (TILs), particularly CD8+ T cells, are associated with a favorable prognosis in breast cancer. B cells produce antibodies that can recognize and neutralize cancer cells. Macrophages within the tumor microenvironment can have both anti-tumor and pro-tumor effects, depending on their polarization. Efforts are underway to enhance the anti-tumor immune response through immunotherapies, including immune checkpoint inhibitors and adoptive cell therapies.

In colon cancer, T cells, particularly CD8+ T cells, are critical for immune surveillance and anti-tumor activity. These T cells infiltrate the tumor and recognize tumor antigens presented by cancer cells. Infiltrating regulatory T cells (Tregs) and myeloid-derived suppressor cells (MDSCs) can suppress the immune response and promote tumor growth. Immune checkpoint molecules, such as PD-1 and CTLA-4, are expressed in colon cancer and their inhibition has shown promise in enhancing T cell-mediated immune responses.

In prostate cancer, the immune system plays a complex role. Prostate tumors can evade immune detection through mechanisms such as downregulation of major histocompatibility complex (MHC) molecules. However, immune cells like T cells, NK cells, and macrophages are still involved in the anti-tumor response. Effector T cells can recognize prostate-specific antigens and infiltrate the tumor to eliminate cancer cells. NK cells also play a role in prostate cancer immune surveillance. Strategies targeting immune checkpoints, such as PD-1 and CTLA-4, have shown promise in activating T cell-mediated immune responses against prostate cancer.

In pancreatic cancer, the immune system faces significant challenges due to the immunosuppressive tumor microenvironment. Tumor-associated macrophages, myeloid-derived suppressor cells (MDSCs), and regulatory T cells (Tregs) contribute to immune suppression. Efforts are underway to overcome these barriers and enhance the anti-tumor immune response. Approaches such as immune checkpoint inhibitors, cancer vaccines, and adoptive cell therapies aim to reinvigorate the immune response against pancreatic cancer cells.

They Lymphatic System as a part of the Immune Network

The lymphatic system is another critical organ in the immune system's fight against cancer. It is a network of vessels and organs that circulate lymph, a clear fluid that contains white blood cells. The lymphatic system works with the immune system to identify and remove foreign invaders, including cancer cells. Lymph nodes, which are small structures located throughout the body, are responsible for filtering lymph and trapping cancer cells. Once cancer cells are trapped in lymph nodes, they are destroyed by immune cells.

In lung cancer, the lymphatic system helps in the removal of cancer cells and facilitates immune surveillance. Lymphatic vessels drain fluid from the lung tissue and transport it to lymph nodes. Cancer cells can travel through lymphatic vessels to regional lymph nodes, where they can be recognized and attacked by immune cells. Lymph nodes contain immune cells, such as lymphocytes, macrophages, and dendritic cells, which help in the detection and elimination of cancer cells. The lymphatic system also plays a role in the dissemination of cancer cells to distant sites, known as metastasis.

In breast cancer, the lymphatic system is closely involved in the spread of cancer cells. Lymphatic vessels in the breast tissue drain fluid, waste products, and cancer cells from the tumor site. Regional lymph nodes, such as the axillary lymph nodes, are often the first sites of cancer cell spread. Examination of these lymph nodes can provide valuable information about the stage and spread of breast cancer. In breast cancer treatment, the status of the lymph nodes is an important consideration for determining the extent of surgery and the need for additional therapies.

In colon cancer, the lymphatic system plays a role in the spread of cancer cells beyond the primary tumor. Lymphatic vessels in the colon drain fluid and cancer cells from the tumor site, transporting them to regional lymph nodes. Lymph nodes serve as filters and contain immune cells that can recognize and attack cancer cells. The presence of cancer cells in the lymph nodes can indicate the potential for further spread and guide treatment decisions. Surgical removal and examination of lymph nodes are commonly performed in colon cancer to determine the extent of the disease.

In prostate cancer, the lymphatic system can be involved in the metastatic spread of cancer cells. Lymphatic vessels drain fluid, waste products, and cancer cells from the prostate gland. Regional lymph nodes, such as the pelvic lymph nodes, are common sites of metastasis in advanced prostate cancer. Imaging techniques and surgical removal of lymph nodes can be used to evaluate the spread of cancer beyond the prostate gland. Lymph nodes also contain immune cells that play a role in immune surveillance and response against prostate cancer cells.

In pancreatic cancer, the lymphatic system is implicated in the dissemination of cancer cells and the formation of distant metastases. Lymphatic vessels in the pancreas transport fluid and cancer cells to regional lymph nodes, where immune cells can recognize and attack the cancer cells. However, pancreatic cancer is often diagnosed at advanced stages when metastasis has occurred. Lymph nodes near the pancreas, such as the celiac and peripancreatic lymph nodes, are commonly affected by metastatic spread. Understanding the involvement of the lymphatic system is important for staging and treatment planning in pancreatic cancer.

The Spleen and The Thymus as a part of the Immune Network

The spleen is another organ that plays a crucial role in the immune system's defense against cancer. It filters blood and removes old or damaged red blood cells, white blood cells, and platelets. The spleen also acts as a reservoir for white blood cells and can release them into the bloodstream in response to infection or inflammation. Meanwhile, the thymus is a gland located behind the breastbone that plays a critical role in the development of T-cells. It produces hormones that stimulate the growth and maturation of T-cells. T-cells that are matured in the thymus are essential for the immune system's ability to identify and destroy cancer cells.

The spleen, located in the upper left abdomen, serves as a filter for blood and plays a crucial role in immune surveillance. In lung cancer, the spleen contributes to the immune response by producing lymphocytes, including T cells and B cells, which are important for recognizing and attacking cancer cells. The spleen also helps in the clearance of damaged or abnormal cells, including cancer cells, from the bloodstream. Additionally, the spleen acts as a reservoir for immune cells and can release them into circulation when needed to fight against cancer cells.

The thymus, located in the upper chest behind the breastbone, is primarily involved in the development and maturation of T cells, which are essential for orchestrating the immune response against cancer cells. In breast cancer, the thymus supports the production and differentiation of T cells that can recognize and target breast cancer cells. The thymus ensures that T cells undergo selection processes to generate a diverse and functional T cell repertoire that can respond to cancer-specific antigens. T cells that recognize and attack cancer cells are then released into circulation to infiltrate the tumor and mount an immune response.

In colon cancer, prostate cancer, and pancreatic cancer, the spleen and thymus also contribute to the immune response against cancer cells. The spleen is involved in producing and activating lymphocytes, including T cells and B cells, which can recognize and eliminate cancer cells in these types of cancer. The thymus plays a critical role in shaping the T cell repertoire and ensuring the generation of T cells capable of recognizing and targeting cancer cells in the colon, prostate, and pancreas.

Furthermore, both the spleen and thymus are involved in immune surveillance, which helps detect and eliminate cancer cells at an early stage. They support the production, activation, and maturation of immune cells that are crucial for mounting an effective anti-tumor immune response.

The Liver and The Lungs as a part of the Immune Network

The liver is another organ that plays a crucial role in the immune system's fight against cancer, including lung cancer, breast cancer, colon cancer, prostate cancer, and pancreatic cancer. The liver is responsible for metabolizing and eliminating cancer-causing agents from the body, it performs several functions related to immunity, including the production of acute-phase proteins and the clearance of toxins and foreign or harmful substances that can potentially lead to cancer development. The liver also produces proteins that are essential for the immune system's function, including complement proteins that can destroy cancer cells.

The lungs are responsible for oxygenating the blood and removing carbon dioxide. They also play a critical role in the immune system's defense against cancer. The lungs are lined with immune cells called alveolar macrophages, which can engulf and destroy cancer cells. The lungs also produce mucus, which can trap cancer cells and prevent them from spreading to other parts of the body.

In lung cancer, the lung plays a critical role in the immune response due to its direct contact with inhaled pathogens and potential cancer cells. The specialized immune cells, alveolar macrophages, act as the first line of defense by engulfing and eliminating foreign substances, including cancer cells. Additionally, the lungs have lymphoid tissue, such as lymph nodes and lymphatic vessels, which support the immune response by filtering and trapping cancer cells that may have spread from the primary tumor.

Furthermore, the liver and lung both have significant interactions with circulating immune cells. The liver contains specialized immune cells called Kupffer cells, which are a type of macrophage responsible for filtering and clearing pathogens, cellular debris, and cancer cells from the blood. These cells play a crucial role in immune surveillance against circulating cancer cells. Similarly, the lung tissue is rich in immune cells, including T cells, B cells, and dendritic cells, which are involved in recognizing and eliminating cancer cells that may have entered the lungs through the bloodstream.

The Skin as a part of the Immune Network

The skin, being the largest organ of the body, plays a vital role in the defense against cancer. Several components of the skin contribute to the fight against cancer cells and help protect against their development and progression.

The outermost layer of the skin, known as the epidermis, serves as a physical barrier that prevents the entry of harmful substances, including carcinogens. The epidermis consists of specialized cells called keratinocytes, which are constantly replenished from the basal layer. These cells undergo a process of differentiation, forming a tough, protective layer that shields underlying tissues from environmental insults. The intact and healthy epidermal barrier is crucial in preventing the penetration and subsequent development of cancer-causing agents.

Within the epidermis, immune cells known as Langerhans cells play a crucial role in the immune surveillance against cancer cells. Langerhans cells are specialized dendritic cells that function as antigen-presenting cells, capturing and presenting antigens, including those from cancer cells, to other immune cells. They initiate and coordinate immune responses by activating T cells, which can recognize and eliminate cancer cells. Langerhans cells also release signaling molecules called cytokines, which stimulate immune cell recruitment and inflammation at the site of potential cancer development.

Additionally, the skin is richly supplied with blood vessels and lymphatic vessels. These vessels allow for the transport of immune cells and molecules, facilitating the immune response against cancer. Lymphatic vessels within the skin help drain fluid and waste products, including cancer cells, from the tissue. Lymph nodes, which receive lymphatic drainage, contain immune cells that can detect and attack cancer cells, playing a crucial role in immune surveillance and defense.

Furthermore, the skin contains melanocytes, specialized cells responsible for producing the pigment melanin. Melanocytes play a critical role in protecting the skin against harmful ultraviolet (UV) radiation from the sun. Exposure to UV radiation can induce DNA damage and increase the risk of skin cancer. Melanocytes produce melanin, which absorbs and dissipates UV radiation, acting as a natural shield against its harmful effects.

The Gut as a part of the Immune Network

The gut, encompassing the gastrointestinal tract, houses several components that contribute to the fight against cancer and help protect against its development and progression.

The intestinal epithelium, lining the inner surface of the gut, acts as a physical barrier against potentially harmful substances, including carcinogens. The epithelial cells form a tightly sealed layer that prevents the entry of pathogens and toxins into the bloodstream. Additionally, the epithelial cells of the gut undergo constant renewal and differentiation, with new cells being generated from the stem cells located in the crypts of Lieberkühn. This constant turnover helps to replace damaged or compromised cells and maintain the integrity of the gut lining.

Meanwhile, the gut can be indirectly connected to the fight

against lung cancer, breast cancer, colon cancer, prostate cancer, and pancreatic cancer through systemic interactions and immune responses.

In lung cancer, the gut components indirectly influence the immune system's response to cancer cells. The gut microbiota, which consists of a diverse community of microorganisms in the gut, plays a crucial role in shaping the systemic immune response. Research suggests that gut microbiota composition can influence the efficacy of immunotherapy in lung cancer. Certain bacteria within the gut microbiota can enhance the response to immunotherapy by promoting anti-tumor immune activity. Modulating the gut microbiota through interventions such as probiotics or fecal microbiota transplantation may hold promise in improving the immune response against lung cancer.

Breast cancer, colon cancer, prostate cancer, and pancreatic cancer primarily originate in tissues distant from the gut. However, the gut components can still have systemic effects on cancer progression. The gut microbiota, for instance, can impact the metabolism and bioavailability of certain drugs used in cancer treatment. It can also influence the immune response and systemic inflammation, which play roles in cancer development and progression. By modulating the gut microbiota, it may be possible to indirectly influence the systemic environment and potentially impact the progression of these cancers.

Additionally, the gut components contribute to systemic immune responses that can influence the progression of various cancers. The gut-associated lymphoid tissue (GALT), located within the gut, contains immune cells that can influence immune surveillance and response against cancer cells throughout the body. These immune cells can migrate from the gut to distant sites and participate in the immune response against cancer cells in lung, breast, colon, prostate, and pancreatic tissues.

The DNA Repair System as a Natural Defense against Cancer

The DNA repair system is a critical mechanism that safeguards the integrity of our genetic material. It plays a vital role in fighting against cancer by identifying and repairing DNA damage that can lead to the development of mutations and, subsequently, cancerous cells. The DNA repair system acts as a surveillance system, constantly monitoring DNA for abnormalities and ensuring its accurate replication and repair.

In general, the DNA repair system protects against cancer by fixing DNA damage caused by various factors, including environmental exposures, chemical agents, radiation, and errors that occur during DNA replication. When DNA damage occurs, specific DNA repair pathways are activated to correct the damage and maintain the stability of the genome. Failure of the DNA repair system can lead to the accumulation of mutations and genomic instability, which are hallmarks of cancer development.

Here are some real examples that highlight the importance of the DNA repair system as a defense against cancer:

1. BRCA1 and BRCA2 mutations in breast and ovarian cancer: Mutations in the BRCA1 and BRCA2 genes are well-known examples of how defects in DNA repair can increase cancer susceptibility. These genes play a critical role in repairing DNA double-strand breaks. In individuals with BRCA1 or BRCA2 mutations, the DNA repair system is compromised, leading to an increased risk of breast and ovarian cancers. These mutations account for a significant proportion of hereditary breast and ovarian cancer cases.

2. Lynch syndrome and colorectal cancer: Lynch syndrome, also known as hereditary nonpolyposis colorectal cancer (HNPCC), is caused by mutations in

DNA mismatch repair (MMR) genes. The MMR system is responsible for correcting errors that occur during DNA replication. In individuals with Lynch syndrome, the DNA repair system is impaired, resulting in an accumulation of mutations and an increased risk of colorectal and other cancers.

3. Xeroderma pigmentosum and skin cancer: Xeroderma pigmentosum (XP) is a rare genetic disorder that affects the ability to repair DNA damage caused by ultraviolet (UV) radiation from the sun. Individuals with XP have mutations in genes involved in nucleotide excision repair (NER), a pathway responsible for repairing UV-induced DNA damage. As a result, they are highly susceptible to skin cancers, including basal cell carcinoma, squamous cell carcinoma, and melanoma.

4. Fanconi anemia and leukemia: Fanconi anemia is an inherited disorder that affects multiple DNA repair pathways, including homologous recombination repair. Patients with Fanconi anemia have a higher risk of developing leukemia and other cancers due to a compromised ability to repair DNA damage.

These examples demonstrate how defects in the DNA repair system can increase the risk of developing specific types of cancer. In the context of most commonly diagnosed cancers, such as lung cancer, breast cancer, colon cancer, prostate cancer, and pancreatic cancer, the DNA repair system plays a crucial role in preventing the accumulation of genetic alterations that can drive tumorigenesis.

For example, in lung cancer, exposure to environmental carcinogens, such as tobacco smoke or certain occupational hazards, can cause DNA damage. The DNA repair system, particularly the nucleotide excision repair pathway, is involved in repairing DNA lesions induced by these carcinogens.

Deficiencies in DNA repair genes, such as those involved in nucleotide excision repair (e.g., XPA, XPC), have been associated with an increased risk of developing lung cancer.

In breast cancer, mutations in genes involved in DNA repair, such as BRCA1 and BRCA2, are well-known risk factors. These genes play a critical role in repairing DNA double-strand breaks, maintaining genomic stability, and suppressing tumor formation. Mutations in these genes compromise the DNA repair system, leading to an increased susceptibility to breast cancer.

Similarly, in colon cancer, defects in DNA repair pathways, such as the mismatch repair (MMR) system, can lead to the accumulation of mutations and the development of colorectal tumors. Hereditary nonpolyposis colorectal cancer (HNPCC), also known as Lynch syndrome, is caused by inherited mutations in MMR genes, which significantly increase the risk of colon and other cancers.

In prostate cancer, defects in DNA repair genes, including BRCA1, BRCA2, and ATM, have been associated with an increased risk of developing aggressive forms of the disease. These DNA repair gene mutations compromise the ability of cells to repair DNA damage, leading to an increased risk of genomic instability and cancer development.

Pancreatic cancer is also characterized by genomic instability and alterations in DNA repair pathways. Mutations in DNA repair genes, such as BRCA2, PALB2, and ATM, have been implicated in familial cases of pancreatic cancer. These mutations impair the ability of cells to repair DNA damage, promoting the accumulation of genetic alterations and the development of pancreatic tumors.

Apoptosis as a Natural Defense against Cancer

Apoptosis, also known as programmed cell death, is a natural defense mechanism against cancer. It is a highly regulated process that eliminates damaged, mutated, or potentially harmful cells to maintain tissue homeostasis and prevent the uncontrolled growth of cancer cells. Here are some real examples that highlight the significance of apoptosis as a defense against cancer:

1. p53 and cell cycle control: The tumor suppressor protein p53 is a key regulator of apoptosis and plays a crucial role in preventing the development of cancer. When cells experience DNA damage or other cellular stresses, p53 is activated, leading to the induction of apoptosis. For example, UV radiation can cause DNA damage in skin cells. In response, p53 triggers apoptosis to eliminate these damaged cells, reducing the risk of skin cancer development.

2. BCL-2 family and mitochondrial apoptosis: The BCL-2 family of proteins regulates the intrinsic or mitochondrial pathway of apoptosis. Some members, such as BAX and BAK, promote apoptosis, while others, like BCL-2 and BCL-xL, inhibit it. Imbalances in the BCL-2 family can contribute to cancer development. For instance, overexpression of anti-apoptotic BCL-2 proteins can promote cell survival and resistance to apoptosis in various cancers, including lymphomas and leukemias.

3. Fas-FasL pathway and immune surveillance: The Fas-FasL pathway is a critical mechanism of apoptosis involved in immune surveillance against cancer cells. When a cell becomes cancerous, it may display abnormal proteins on its surface. Immune cells, such as cytotoxic T lymphocytes (CTLs), recognize these abnormalities and initiate apoptosis by binding to the Fas receptor on the cancer cell, triggering a cascade of events that leads to cell death. Defects in the Fas-FasL pathway can compromise immune surveillance and

increase the risk of cancer development.

4. Tumor necrosis factor (TNF) and immune-mediated apoptosis: TNF is a cytokine that plays a crucial role in immune responses, including the induction of apoptosis. It can directly trigger apoptosis in cancer cells by binding to TNF receptors on their surface. Additionally, TNF can activate immune cells, such as macrophages, to produce other molecules that promote apoptosis in cancer cells. TNF-based therapies, such as TNF-alpha inhibitors, have been developed to target specific cancers, such as certain types of lymphomas and sarcomas.

These examples illustrate how apoptosis acts as a natural defense against cancer by eliminating damaged or abnormal cells. Apoptosis prevents the propagation of cells with genomic alterations, inhibits the survival of cancer cells, and enhances immune-mediated destruction of cancerous cells. Dysregulation of apoptosis can contribute to cancer development by allowing the survival and proliferation of abnormal cells.

In lung cancer, apoptosis is disrupted due to genetic alterations and dysregulation of key apoptotic pathways. For instance, mutations in the tumor suppressor gene TP53 (p53) are common in lung cancer and can impair apoptosis. p53 regulates the expression of pro-apoptotic genes, and its dysfunction contributes to the survival and proliferation of lung cancer cells.

In breast cancer, apoptosis plays a crucial role in breast cancer development and treatment response. Defective apoptotic pathways can contribute to the resistance of breast cancer cells to chemotherapy and targeted therapies. Understanding the molecular mechanisms of apoptosis in breast cancer is crucial for identifying novel therapeutic strategies to induce apoptosis and improve treatment outcomes.

In colon cancer, apoptosis dysregulation is implicated in the development of colon cancer. Mutations in the adenomatous polyposis coli (APC) gene, a tumor suppressor gene commonly associated with colon cancer, can disrupt apoptosis. Dysfunctional apoptosis pathways allow the survival and proliferation of abnormal cells, contributing to the formation of colon tumors.

In prostate cancer, apoptosis resistance is a hallmark of prostate cancer progression and treatment resistance. Prostate cancer cells can acquire alterations that allow them to evade apoptosis, leading to uncontrolled growth. Targeting apoptotic pathways, such as the BCL-2 family proteins, is being explored as a potential therapeutic approach to induce apoptosis in prostate cancer cells.

In pancreatic cancer, apoptosis evasion is a characteristic feature of pancreatic cancer. Genetic alterations and dysregulation of apoptotic pathways contribute to the survival and proliferation of pancreatic cancer cells. Understanding the molecular mechanisms underlying apoptosis resistance in pancreatic cancer is crucial for developing effective treatment strategies.

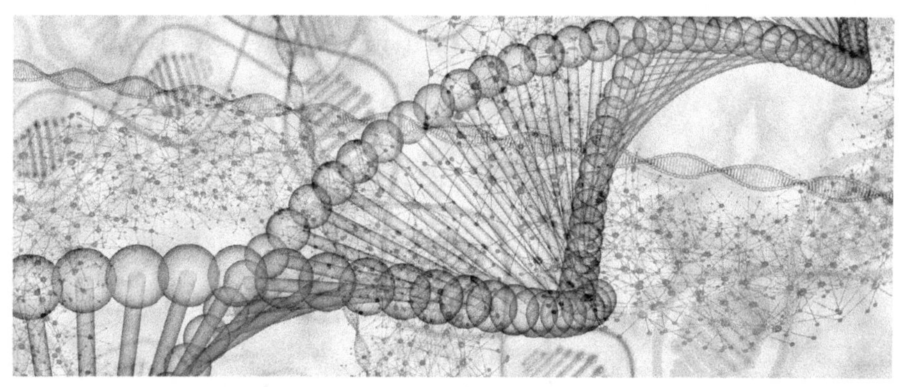

CHAPTER 3 WHEN CANCER BECOME DEADLY: BENIGN VS MALIGNANT TUMORS

Cancer and tumor are not necessarily the same thing. A tumor is an abnormal growth of cells that can be benign or malignant. Benign tumors, unlike malignant tumors, do not spread to other parts of the body and are not life-threatening; while cancers are malignant tumors that are life-threatening. However, even benign tumors can cause health problems if they grow large enough or put pressure on surrounding tissues. In this chapter, we will review both benign tumors and malignant tumors aka. deadly cancers.

Benign Tumors are not Cancer

Benign tumors can develop in any part of the body, including the brain, lungs, breast, liver, and skin. Some of the most common types of benign tumors include:

Benign Tumor Type	Brief Description	Average Occurrence Age
Adenomas	Noncancerous	50s-60s

	growths that form in the glandular tissue of organs such as the colon, thyroid, pituitary gland and liver	
Lipomas	Soft, rubbery growths that form under the skin and are made up of fat cells, most commonly found in the neck, shoulders, and back	40s-60s
Fibromas	Noncancerous growths that form in the fibrous tissue of organs such as the uterus, skin, and breasts	20s-40s
Meningiomas	Noncancerous tumors that form in the membranes that cover the brain and spinal cord	40s-70s
Ovarian cysts	Fluid-filled sacs that form on or within the ovaries	30s-50s
Uterine fibroids	Noncancerous growths that form in the muscular tissue of the uterus	30s-50s
Hemangiomas	Benign tumors made up of blood vessels that usually form on the skin, liver or brain	Birth to 1 year

Papillomas	Noncancerous growths that form in the skin or mucous membranes, often causing warts or polyps	30s-50s
Nevus (Mole)	A type of pigmented skin lesion that can vary in size, color, and shape	Birth to 30s
Thyroid nodules	Noncancerous growths that form in the thyroid gland and can sometimes be felt as a lump in the neck	30s-50s

The exact cause of benign tumors is not always known, but some factors that may increase the risk of developing a benign tumor include: a) Genetic mutations: Changes in certain genes can cause cells to grow and divide uncontrollably, leading to the development of a tumor; b) Hormonal imbalances: Hormonal imbalances, such as those that occur during pregnancy or menopause, can increase the risk of developing certain types of benign tumors;   c) Exposure to radiation: Exposure to high levels of radiation can increase the risk of developing a benign tumor; d) Immune system disorders: Certain immune system disorders, such as lupus, can increase the risk of developing a benign tumor.

The symptoms of a benign tumor vary depending on its location and size. Some common symptoms include: a lump or mass that can be felt under the skin; pain or discomfort in the affected area; changes in bowel or bladder habits; headaches or seizures in the case of a brain tumor; changes in vision or hearing etc. To diagnose a benign tumor, a doctor may perform various tests, including imaging tests such as X-rays, CT scans, and MRI scans; biopsy removed from the tumor to be examined under a microscope; blood tests to identify any hormonal imbalances that may be causing the tumor.

Treatment of a Benign Tumor

The treatment of a benign tumor depends on its location and size, as well as the symptoms it is causing. Some common treatment options include:

Treatment Option	Brief Description	Typical Treatment Cycle
Watchful Waiting	Monitoring the tumor for any changes or growth over time, with no immediate intervention	Regular check-ups or imaging scans, often every 3-6 months
Surgery	Removing the tumor through a surgical procedure	Usually a one-time procedure, although some larger or complex tumors may require multiple surgeries
Radiation Therapy	Using high-energy radiation to shrink or destroy the tumor cells	Several weeks of daily treatments, often 5 days a week
Hormone Therapy	Using medications or hormone-blocking drugs to slow or stop the growth of hormone-sensitive tumors	Daily or periodic doses, often for several months or years
Embolization	Blocking the blood vessels that supply the tumor with blood and nutrients, causing it to shrink or die	Typically a one-time procedure, but may require follow-up treatments
Cryotherapy	Freezing the tumor cells with extreme cold	Typically a one-time procedure, but may

temperatures, causing them to die off	require follow-up treatments

Malignant Tumors are Cancer

In contrast, malignant tumors, or cancer will become deadly when it grows and spreads uncontrollably, invading nearby tissues and organs, and potentially spreading to other parts of the body through a process known as metastasis. At this point, cancer cells can break away from the primary tumor and travel through the bloodstream or lymphatic system to other parts of the body, form new tumors, making the cancer more difficult to treat and reducing the chances of survival. The prognosis of cancer depends on several factors, including the type and stage of cancer, the patient's age and overall health, and the effectiveness of the treatment. In general, cancer is more likely to be deadly if it is detected at a later stage, as it may have already spread to other parts of the body, making it more difficult to treat. The five-year survival rate is a commonly used statistic to describe the percentage of patients who are alive five years after being diagnosed with cancer. For example, the five-year survival rate for breast cancer is around 90% when the cancer is detected early and has not spread to other parts of the body. However, if the cancer has spread to distant parts of the body, the five-year survival rate drops to around 28%. The 5-year survival rate for cancer can provide important information for patients and their families, but it is important to remember that it is just one factor in determining the prognosis for cancer patients. The rate can vary widely depending on the type and stage of cancer, as well as other factors such as the patient's age and overall health.

Another commonly used term is "5-year survival rate by stage of cancer", which uses the stage of cancer at the point of diagnosis when calculating survival. Although simplified classification of either local cancer or metastatic cancer is useful, a more thorough definition of stages are as follows:

- stage 1 cancer (small and localized)
- stage 2 cancer (larger bust still localized)
- stage 3 cancer (spread to surrounding tissues or lymph nodes)
- stage 4 cancer (spread to other parts of the body)

In Figure shown below, based on SEER data submission (https://seer.cancer/gov), we can see that for the eight most common types of solid tumors, despite significant progress made against cancer, the progress has not been uniform for all types and stages of cancer at diagnosis. In all cases, the 5-year survival rate is substantially lower for those diagnosed with stage 3 or stage 4 cancers which has spread to distant sites.

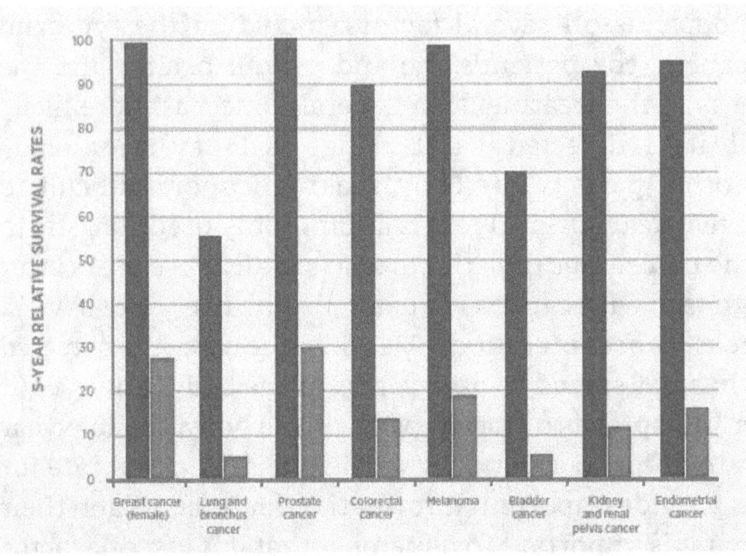

Metastatic Cancer

Not surprisingly, metastatic cancer is much more difficult to treat than cancer that is confined to one area of the body, and it is responsible for the majority of cancer-related deaths. The top 5 cancer types that cause the most deaths in the US are:

1) Lung cancer: Lung cancer is the leading cause of cancer-related deaths in the US, accounting for about 23% of all cancer deaths. Smoking is the primary cause of lung cancer,

but exposure to secondhand smoke, air pollution, and certain occupational hazards can also increase the risk.

2) Colorectal cancer: Colorectal cancer is the second leading cause of cancer-related deaths in the US, accounting for about 9% of all cancer deaths. The risk of colorectal cancer increases with age and is influenced by factors such as a family history of the disease, a diet high in red and processed meats, and a sedentary lifestyle.

3) Breast cancer: Breast cancer is the third leading cause of cancer-related deaths in the US, accounting for about 7% of all cancer deaths. While breast cancer can occur in both men and women, it is much more common in women. Factors that can increase the risk of breast cancer include a family history of the disease, exposure to estrogen, and certain genetic mutations.

4) Pancreatic cancer: Pancreatic cancer is the fourth leading cause of cancer-related deaths in the US, accounting for about 7% of all cancer deaths. It is one of the most deadly forms of cancer, as it is often diagnosed at an advanced stage when it has already spread to other parts of the body. Smoking, obesity, and a family history of pancreatic cancer can increase the risk.

5) Prostate cancer: Prostate cancer is the fifth leading cause of cancer-related deaths in the US, accounting for about 5% of all cancer deaths. It is most common in men over the age of 50, and the risk increases with age. Factors that can increase the risk of prostate cancer include a family history of the disease, African American race, and exposure to certain chemicals.

When someone is dying of metastatic cancer, it can be due to a variety of factors. With metastatic cancer spreading from its original site to other parts of the body, this spread can cause damage to organs and tissues, which can ultimately lead to organ failure. For example, if cancer spreads to the liver, it can cause liver failure, which can be fatal. Similarly, if cancer spreads to the lungs, it can cause respiratory failure. However, the causes of death in someone with metastatic cancer can also include complications related to the cancer itself or its treatment.

In addition to organ failure, there are several other causes of death in someone with metastatic cancer. These can include infections, blood clots, and complications related to the cancer treatment itself, such as chemotherapy-induced toxicity or radiation-induced damage.

Pain and other symptoms related to cancer can also contribute to a decline in quality of life in someone with metastatic cancer. For example, if cancer has spread to the bones, it can cause pain and make it difficult to move or perform daily activities. Similarly, if cancer has spread to the brain, it can cause neurological symptoms such as seizures or confusion.

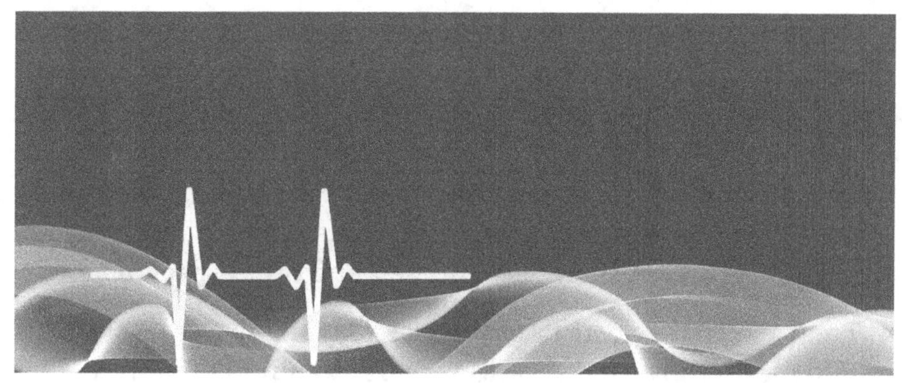

SECTION II UNDERSTANDING SIX MAJOR OPTIONS FOR CANCER TREATMENT

Although there are more than 100 types of cancer and related hereditary syndromes, the process of diagnosing and treating different cancers tends to be similar, typically involving several steps and a multidisciplinary team of healthcare professionals.

Process of Diagnosing and Treating a Cancer

Here is an overview of the process:

1. Initial diagnosis: Cancer may be suspected based on a patient's symptoms or abnormal test results. A healthcare provider may perform a physical exam, review the patient's medical history, and order imaging tests or laboratory tests such as blood tests or biopsies to confirm the diagnosis.

2. Staging: Once cancer is confirmed, the extent and stage of the cancer are determined through various imaging tests such as CT scans, MRI, PET scans, or bone scans. The stage of cancer helps determine the appropriate treatment plan.

3. Treatment decision: The treatment decision is based on the type, stage, and location of cancer, as well as the patient's overall health and preferences. The treatment plan may involve surgery, radiation therapy, chemotherapy, immunotherapy, or a combination of these treatments. The treatment team may include various healthcare professionals such as oncologists, surgeons, radiation therapists, nurses, and other specialists.

4. Treatment: The treatment process may involve several cycles of chemotherapy or radiation therapy, surgical removal of the tumor or affected tissue, or immunotherapy to boost the immune system to fight cancer cells.

5. Follow-up: After completing the initial treatment, patients may need to undergo periodic imaging tests or laboratory tests to monitor for any recurrence or progression of cancer. Follow-up care also includes addressing any side effects of the treatment and providing supportive care.

Throughout the diagnostic and treatment process, various tests and imaging may be performed depending on the type and stage of cancer. Some of the commonly used tests and imaging include:

1) Biopsy: A sample of the tumor or affected tissue is removed and examined under a microscope by a pathologist to determine the type and stage of cancer.

2) Imaging tests: CT scans, MRI, PET scans, or bone scans are used to visualize the location and extent of cancer.

3) Blood tests: Blood tests may be used to detect cancer markers, such as PSA for prostate cancer or CA-125 for ovarian cancer.

4) Endoscopy: A flexible tube with a camera is inserted through the mouth or rectum to visualize the affected area and take tissue samples.

5) Genetic testing: Genetic testing may be performed to determine if a patient has an inherited predisposition to certain

types of cancer, or mutation biomarkers suitable for targeted therapy or immunotherapy.

The lead on a cancer patient's treatment team may vary depending on the type and stage of cancer and the treatment plan. In general, the oncologist is often the lead on the treatment team and works closely with other healthcare professionals to provide coordinated care. However, the treatment team may also include surgeons, radiation therapists, nurses, and other specialists who work together to develop and implement the treatment plan.

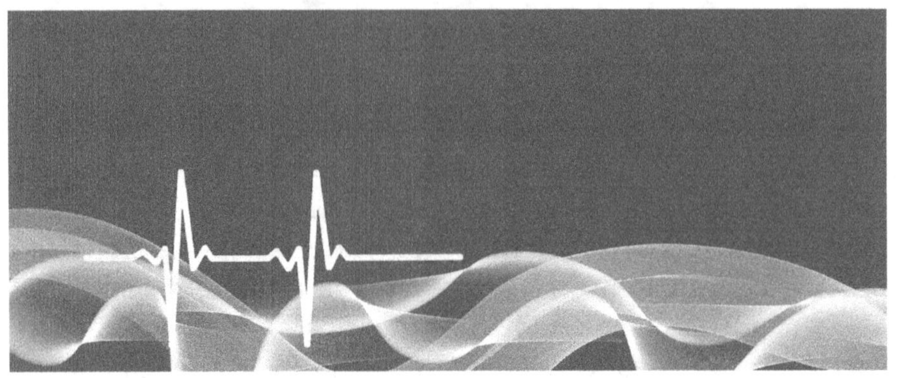

CHAPTER 4 SURGERY AS A CANCER TREATMENT OPTION

Surgery has been a cornerstone of medical practice since ancient times. The first surgical procedures were crude and often performed without anesthesia or antiseptic techniques, resulting in high mortality rates. Over the years, surgical techniques and technologies have continued to advance, leading to improved outcomes and better patient care. In recent years, there have been exciting developments in surgery, including the use of minimally invasive techniques, robotic surgery, and image-guided surgery. These advances have allowed for more precise and targeted surgical interventions, leading to faster recovery times, reduced pain and scarring, and improved overall patient outcomes.

In the field of cancer treatment, surgery plays a critical role in the management of many types of cancer, including lung cancer, breast cancer, colon cancer, and pancreatic cancer. Surgical removal of tumors and affected tissues is often a key component of cancer treatment. Advances in surgical techniques have allowed for the removal of tumors with greater precision and reduced morbidity, leading to improved survival rates and quality of life for cancer patients. In addition, the use of advanced imaging techniques, such as MRI and PET scans, has allowed for more accurate mapping of tumor location and growth, enabling surgeons to perform more precise and targeted surgeries. Other recent developments, such as the use of intraoperative radiation therapy and the development of new surgical tools, have also had a significant impact on cancer treatment.

Let's look at a patient's success story with cancer surgery: Sally Smith in New York was diagnosed with Stage II breast cancer at age of 54 in 2019 during a routine mammogram. Her doctor recommended a lumpectomy followed by radiation therapy. Sally was nervous about undergoing surgery, but her doctor explained the benefits of the procedure and answered all of her questions. The surgery was performed in early 2020 and was successful in removing the cancerous tumor. Sally was able to return to her normal activities within a few weeks after surgery. She then underwent radiation therapy as planned and completed her treatment in the summer of 2020. Today, Sally is cancer-free and is grateful for the care and support she received from her medical team. She encourages all women to get regular mammograms and to trust their doctors if they are diagnosed with breast cancer.

It is important to note that minimally invasive surgeries, such as laparoscopic and robotic surgeries, are becoming more common for many types of cancer surgery, but some cancers or advanced cases may still require open surgery. Here are the surgery options for a few of the most common cancers.

A) Lung Cancer Surgery

Here is a table showing the most common types of lung cancer surgeries, their percentage of procedures, and a brief description of each option:

Surgery Type	Percentage of Procedures	Description
Lobectomy	50-60%	Removal of the lobe of the lung that contains the tumor
Pneumonectomy	10-15%	Removal of the entire lung that contains the tumor
Segmentectomy	5-10%	Removal of a smaller part of the lung that contains the tumor
Wedge Resection	10-15%	Removal of the tumor and a small margin of healthy tissue
Sleeve Resection	<5%	Removal of a section of the bronchus that contains the tumor and reattachment of the remaining sections of the bronchus

Video-assisted thoracoscopic surgery (VATS) is a minimally invasive surgical technique used to diagnose and treat conditions of the chest, including lung cancer. The procedure involves making several small incisions in the chest and inserting a thoracoscope, a small camera connected to a video monitor, which allows the surgeon to see inside the chest cavity without making a large incision.

During VATS lung cancer surgery, the surgeon uses specialized instruments to remove the cancerous tissue from the lung. The procedure is guided by the images from the thoracoscope, which provides a clear view of the lung and surrounding tissue.

VATS has become increasingly popular in recent years and is now considered the standard of care for many types of lung cancer surgery. In fact, studies have shown that VATS allows for a more precise and targeted removal of the cancerous tissue while minimizing damage to healthy lung tissue, results in better outcomes for patients, including lower rates of complications, shorter hospital stays, and lower healthcare costs.

VATS is particularly useful for early-stage lung cancer, as it allows for precise removal of the cancerous tissue while preserving as much of the healthy lung tissue as possible. It is also being used in more complex cases, including cases where the cancer has spread to other parts of the chest. In these cases, VATS can be combined with other treatment modalities, such as chemotherapy and radiation therapy, to provide a comprehensive approach to cancer treatment.

Robotic-assisted surgery is the fastest-growing kind of surgery for lung cancer. It has all the benefits of minimally invasive VATS. During the surgery, the robot is controlled by a surgeon who uses a console with hand and foot controls to maneuver the robot's arms and instruments. The robot provides a 3D view of the surgical site, which allows the surgeon to operate with greater precision and accuracy.

The benefits of robot-assisted surgery for lung cancer include:

1. Reduced blood loss: Because the incisions are smaller and the surgical robot provides a more precise tool, there is less blood loss during the operation.

2. Shorter hospital stays: Patients who undergo robot-assisted surgery typically spend less time in the hospital, with an average stay of 2-3 days.

3. Faster recovery: The smaller incisions and reduced trauma to the surrounding tissue allow for a faster recovery time and less post-operative pain.

4. Improved outcomes: Studies have shown that robot-

assisted surgery can lead to better outcomes and lower complication rates compared to traditional open surgery.

For example, Memorial Sloan Kettering Cancer Center (MSKCC) does more than 440 minimally invasive lung cancer surgeries each year, with VATS used with nearly 6 out of 10 patients, making it one of the busiest cancer centers for these procedures.

B) Breast Cancer Surgery

The most common choice for breast cancer surgery depends on several factors, including the size and location of the tumor, the stage of the cancer, and the patient's personal preferences. In general, lumpectomy is preferred if the tumor is small and the cancer has not spread, while mastectomy may be necessary if the tumor is large or if there is a high risk of recurrence. Here's a table showing different options for breast cancer surgery, their percentage of use, and a brief description:

Breast Cancer Surgery Option	Percentage of Use	Description
Lumpectomy	60%	Removal of only the tumor and a small amount of surrounding tissue, while preserving the majority of the breast tissue
Mastectomy	38%	Removal of the entire breast
Unilateral Mastectomy	24%	Removal of the affected breast only
Bilateral Mastectomy	14%	Removal of both breasts

Double Mastectomy with Reconstruction	2%	Removal of both breasts followed by immediate breast reconstruction

Many women with early-stage cancers can choose between having lumpectomy (or breast conversing surgery, BCS) and mastectomy. The main advantage of BCS is that a woman keeps most of her breast. But most often, she will also need radiation. Women who have mastectomy for early-stage cancers are less likely to need radiation.

For some women, mastectomy may be a better option or the only option, because of the type of breast cancer, the large size of the tumor, previous treatment with radiation, or certain other factors.

Some women might worry that having a less extensive surgery might raise the risk of the cancer coming back. But studies of thousands of women over more than 20 years show that when BCS is done with radiation, survival is the same as having a mastectomy, in people with early-stage cancer who are candidates for both types of surgery.

While mastectomy involves removing the entire breast, there are several types of mastectomies, including:

- Simple mastectomy: This involves removing the breast tissue but not the lymph nodes or muscle.

- Modified radical mastectomy: This involves removing the breast tissue, some of the lymph nodes, and the lining over the chest muscles.

- Radical mastectomy: This involves removing the entire breast, the lymph nodes, and the chest muscles.

Breast cancer surgery has seen significant advancements in

recent years with the introduction of new surgical options that aim to provide improved cosmetic outcomes, minimize morbidity, and maximize survival rates. Here are some of the newest surgical options available in breast cancer surgery:

1. Nipple-sparing mastectomy (NSM): NSM is a surgical technique that preserves the nipple and areola while removing the breast tissue. NSM is an option for women with small tumors and those who are at low risk of developing breast cancer in the nipple.

2. Oncoplastic surgery: This technique combines the principles of plastic surgery with breast cancer surgery. Oncoplastic surgery aims to remove the cancer while preserving the breast shape and contour. It can be performed as a single procedure or in multiple stages, depending on the size and location of the tumor.

3. Hidden Scar surgery: This technique involves making incisions in inconspicuous areas of the breast, such as along the natural creases or the edge of the areola. This technique aims to minimize scarring and improve cosmetic outcomes.

4. Intraoperative radiation therapy (IORT): IORT involves delivering a single dose of radiation therapy to the tumor bed during surgery. This technique aims to reduce radiation exposure to healthy tissues and decrease the duration of treatment.

5. Sentinel lymph node biopsy (SLNB): SLNB is a minimally invasive procedure that involves removing only the lymph nodes that are most likely to contain cancer cells. This technique aims to reduce the risk of complications associated with the removal of all axillary lymph nodes.

These surgical options have several benefits, including reduced scarring, faster recovery, improved cosmetic outcomes, and reduced risk of complications. However, post-surgical care is still important, and patients need to follow their surgeon's instructions carefully to ensure proper healing and recovery. Patients may need to wear a compression garment, avoid heavy lifting, and perform specific exercises to promote healing and reduce the risk of complications such as lymphedema.

C) Colon Cancer Surgery

When colon cancer is found early, the tumor is often fully contained within an abnormal growth on the inside lining of the colon. This is called a polyp. Removing a polyp during a colonoscopy may be enough to cure the cancer. When colon cancer has begun to spread through the colon, more extensive surgeries would be needed. Surgery is the main treatment for colon cancer, and the type of surgery performed depends on the stage and location of the cancer. Here's a table of common colon cancer surgery options, their approximate percentage of use, and a brief description of each option:

Surgery Option	Percentage of Procedures	Description
Colectomy	55-65%	Removal of a portion of the colon affected by cancer, along with surrounding lymph nodes. The two ends of the remaining colon are then reattached.
Laparoscopic Colectomy	25-35%	A minimally invasive procedure where small incisions are made and a laparoscope and specialized instruments are used to remove the affected portion of the colon.
Robotic Colectomy	5-10%	Similar to laparoscopic colectomy, but a robotic arm is used to control the instruments.

Abdominoperineal Resection	5-10%	A more extensive surgery used for rectal cancer, where the rectum, anus, and surrounding tissue are removed, and the end of the colon is brought out to the abdominal wall to form a permanent colostomy.
Local Excision	1-2%	Removal of small, early-stage tumors in the colon wall, performed through the anus without major incisions.
Total Colectomy	<1%	Removal of the entire colon, sometimes performed in cases of inherited colorectal cancer syndromes or extensive disease. A colostomy bag is needed to collect waste.

For newly diagnosed colon cancer patients, one of the first concerns that many patients have is whether they will need to use a colostomy bag. Depending on the stage and location of the cancer, most patients with colon cancer do not need a colostomy bag. If you do, it is usually reversed after a short time. After the two ends of the colon are surgically reconnected, you can go back to your normal bathroom habits.

D) Prostate Cancer Surgery

Here is a table showing the most common types of prostate cancer surgeries, their percentage of procedures, and a brief description of each option:

Surgery Type	Percentage of Procedures	Description
Radical Prostatectomy	60%	Surgical removal of the prostate gland and some surrounding tissues. Can be done as open surgery or minimally invasive laparoscopic or robotic-assisted surgery.
Transurethral Resection of the Prostate (TURP)	12%	Removal of part of the prostate gland through the urethra using a resectoscope. Often used for benign prostatic hyperplasia (BPH) but can also be used for early stage prostate cancer.
Cryosurgery	4%	Freezing of the prostate gland to destroy cancer cells. Can be done as a minimally invasive procedure using needles inserted through the skin or transrectally.
High-Intensity Focused Ultrasound (HIFU)	3%	Use of high-frequency ultrasound waves to heat and destroy cancer cells in the prostate gland. Can be done as a minimally invasive procedure.
Radiation Therapy	21%	Use of high-energy radiation to destroy cancer cells in the prostate gland. Can be done as external beam radiation therapy or brachytherapy (radioactive seeds implanted in the prostate gland).

		Monitoring of the cancer with regular PSA tests, digital rectal exams, and prostate biopsies. Treatment is deferred until there are signs of cancer
Active Surveillance	16%	progression.

As mentioned earlier, with minimally invasive surgery, a patient is likely to have less discomfort after the procedure and more likely to recover faster than with a traditional open surgery. Many men who have their prostates removed in a minimally invasive operation with experienced surgeons are able to return home the following day.

E) Pancreatic Cancer Surgery

Here is a table showing the most common types of pancreatic cancer surgeries, their percentage of procedures, and a brief description of each option:

Surgery Type	Percentage of Procedures	Description
Whipple Procedure	80%	This surgery involves removing the head of the pancreas, the duodenum, a portion of the stomach, and the gallbladder. In some cases, the bile duct may also be

		removed. This procedure is the most common surgery for pancreatic cancer.
Distal Pancreatectomy	10%	This surgery involves removing the tail of the pancreas and sometimes the body of the pancreas. The spleen may also be removed. This surgery is typically used for tumors located in the tail of the pancreas.
Total Pancreatectomy	5%	This surgery involves removing the entire pancreas, part of the stomach, part of the small intestine, the common

		bile duct, the gallbladder, the spleen, and nearby lymph nodes. This surgery is used for patients with tumors that have spread throughout the pancreas.
Laparoscopic Surgery	5%	This type of surgery involves making several small incisions in the abdomen and using a laparoscope to remove the tumor. This surgery may be used for smaller tumors that have not spread to nearby tissues.

There have been several recent developments in pancreatic cancer surgery aimed at improving patient outcomes and reducing side effects. Some of these include:

1. Robotic-assisted surgery: Like in other types of cancer surgeries, robotic-assisted surgery is becoming more common in pancreatic cancer surgery. This approach can help improve precision and reduce recovery time.

2. Neoadjuvant therapy: This refers to chemotherapy or radiation therapy given before surgery. Studies have shown that neoadjuvant therapy can help shrink tumors, making them easier to remove during surgery.

3. Laparoscopic surgery: This approach uses small incisions and a tiny camera to guide the surgeon. Compared to open surgery, laparoscopic surgery can result in less blood loss, less pain, and a faster recovery.

4. Enhanced recovery after surgery (ERAS) protocols: These protocols involve a coordinated approach to surgery and recovery that can help patients return to their normal activities more quickly. They typically involve steps such as early feeding after surgery and early mobilization.

5. Targeted therapies: These are drugs that specifically target cancer cells, often in combination with surgery. For example, some targeted therapies may help shrink tumors before surgery, making them easier to remove.

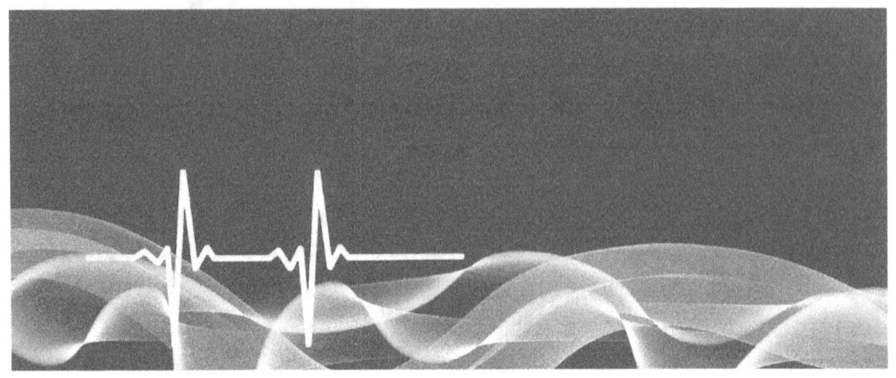

CHAPTER 5 RADIATION THERAPY AS A CANCER TREATMENT OPTION

Radiation therapy is a common form of cancer treatment that uses high-energy radiation to kill cancer cells and shrink tumors. Radiation therapy is most effective in treating localized cancers, such as those found in the prostate, lung, and breast. Radiation therapy works by damaging the DNA inside cancer cells, which stops them from dividing and growing. The radiation can be delivered to the cancer cells in different ways, including external beam radiation and internal radiation (brachytherapy).

External beam radiation therapy is the most common type of radiation therapy. It uses a machine called a linear accelerator to deliver high-energy radiation beams to the cancer cells from outside the body. The radiation is carefully aimed at the cancer cells to minimize damage to healthy tissue.

Internal radiation therapy, or brachytherapy, involves placing a radioactive source directly into or near the cancerous tissue. This type of radiation therapy is commonly used for certain types of cancer, such as prostate cancer or gynecological cancers.

Radiation therapy is usually given in multiple sessions over a period of several weeks. Each session is relatively quick and painless, usually taking only a few minutes. Side effects of radiation therapy can include fatigue, skin changes, and irritation of the treated area. These side effects are usually temporary and can be managed with medication and other therapies.

Let's look at a cancer patient's success story with radiation therapy: John Smith was diagnosed with prostate cancer at the age of 62. His urologist recommended radiation therapy as the primary treatment option. John was referred to a radiation oncologist who recommended a course of external beam radiation therapy (EBRT) over the course of eight weeks. John underwent daily treatments, five days a week.

During the course of treatment, John experienced some mild fatigue and skin irritation in the treated area, but overall, he tolerated the treatment well. After completing the treatment, John's PSA levels began to decrease, and his cancer was considered to be in remission.

Several years later, John's PSA levels began to rise again, indicating a possible recurrence of his cancer. His radiation oncologist recommended a course of salvage radiation therapy, which is radiation given after an initial treatment has failed. John underwent another eight-week course of EBRT and was once again able to achieve remission.

John is now 76 years old, and his cancer has not returned. He continues to see his radiation oncologist regularly for follow-up appointments and PSA monitoring.

Variety of Radiation Therapy Available

Radiation therapy is often used in combination with other treatments, such as surgery or chemotherapy, to improve outcomes for patients. Here is a table showing radiation therapy options for cancer patients, their percentage of procedures, and a brief description of each option:

Radiation Therapy Option	Percentage of Procedures	Brief Description	Pros	Cons
External Beam Radiation Therapy (EBRT)	65%	Uses high-energy beams from a machine outside the body to target cancer cells. The treatment is typically given 5 days a week for several weeks.	Non-invasive, effective for localized tumors.	Long treatment time, risk of radiation exposure to surrounding tissues.
Intensity-Modulated Radiation Therapy (IMRT)	20%	Advanced form of EBRT that uses computer-controlled beams of radiation to precisely target the tumor.	Higher accuracy, reduces radiation exposure to healthy tissues.	Longer treatment time, more expensive than conventional radiation therapy.
Proton Therapy	5%	Uses protons instead of x-rays to deliver radiation to the cancer cells. This allows for higher doses to be delivered to the tumor while	Minimizes radiation exposure to healthy tissues, effective for hard-to-reach tumors.	Limited availability, high cost.

		sparing surrounding healthy tissue.		
Brachytherapy	5%	Involves placing radioactive sources directly into or near the cancerous tissue. This can be done through implants, injections, or through applicators temporarily placed in the body.	Minimizes radiation exposure to healthy tissues, precise delivery of radiation.	Only suitable for certain types of cancers and locations, may require hospitalization.
Stereotactic Radiosurgery (SRS)	5%	Delivers high-dose radiation to a precise area of the body in one or a few treatments. It is commonly used for brain tumors or small lung tumors.	Non-invasive, effective for small, hard-to-reach tumors.	May cause swelling or damage to surrounding tissues, not suitable for large tumors.

Intraoperative Radiation Therapy (IORT): Delivers a single, high dose of radiation to the tumor during surgery. It can be used for a variety of cancers, including breast and pancreatic cancer.

Recent advances in radiation therapy have allowed for more precise targeting of cancer cells, reducing damage to healthy tissue and improving treatment outcomes.

One of the most significant recent developments in radiation therapy is the use of intensity-modulated radiation therapy (IMRT). This technology allows for precise control of the radiation beam intensity, allowing for greater targeting of cancer cells and reduced exposure to healthy tissue. IMRT has been shown to be effective in treating a variety of cancers, including prostate, head and neck, and breast cancers.

Another important advance in radiation therapy is the use of stereotactic body radiation therapy (SBRT), also known as stereotactic ablative radiation therapy (SABR). SBRT uses highly focused radiation beams to deliver high doses of radiation to small, well-defined tumors, such as those found in the lungs or liver. SBRT has been shown to be highly effective in treating early-stage lung cancer and is being increasingly used for other types of cancer.

In addition to IMRT and SBRT, other advanced radiation therapy techniques include proton therapy, which uses a beam of protons to deliver radiation to the tumor, and brachytherapy, which involves placing small, radioactive seeds directly into the tumor or near it. These techniques are often used for specific types of cancer, such as prostate or gynecologic cancers.

Radiation Therapy Usage in Treating Lung Cancer, Breast Cancer, Colon Cancer, Prostate Cancer and Pancreatic Cancer

Finally, here's a table showing how radiation therapy is used in the treatment of early and advanced stage lung cancer, breast cancer, colon cancer, prostate cancer, and pancreatic cancer:

Cancer Type	Early Stage	Advanced Stage
Lung Cancer	Used alone or in combination with surgery and/or chemotherapy, or as a primary treatment for patients who are	Used palliatively to relieve symptoms and improve quality of life

	not candidates for surgery	
Breast Cancer	Used after breast-conserving surgery or mastectomy to destroy remaining cancer cells	Used to relieve symptoms and improve quality of life in advanced stage or metastatic breast cancer
Colon Cancer	Used after surgery to destroy any remaining cancer cells	Used palliatively to relieve symptoms and improve quality of life in advanced stage or metastatic colon cancer
Prostate Cancer	Used after surgery or in combination with hormone therapy to destroy remaining cancer cells, may be used as a primary treatment for patients with early-stage prostate cancer	Used to relieve symptoms and improve quality of life in advanced stage or metastatic prostate cancer
Pancreatic Cancer	Used in combination with chemotherapy to shrink tumors before surgery or as a primary treatment for patients who are not candidates for surgery	Used palliatively to relieve symptoms and improve quality of life in advanced stage or metastatic pancreatic cancer

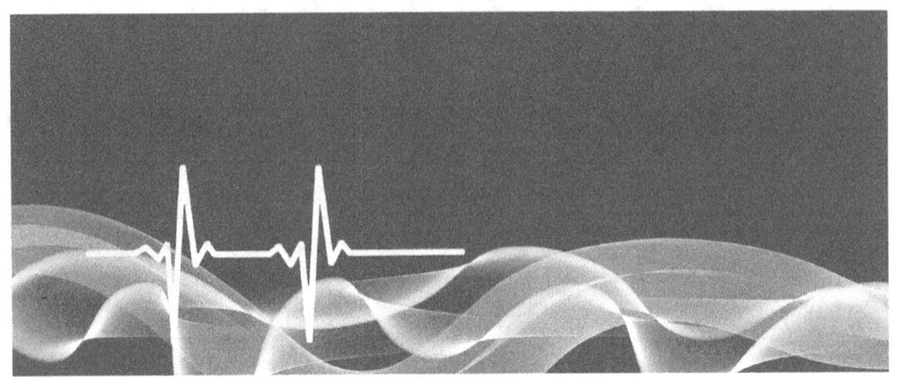

CHAPTER 6 CHEMOTHERAPY AS
A CANCER TREATMENT OPTION

Chemotherapy is a type of cancer treatment that uses drugs to kill cancer cells or stop them from growing and multiplying. It is one of the most widely used treatments for cancer and has been in use since the 1940s.

The drugs used in chemotherapy work by attacking cells that are rapidly dividing, such as cancer cells. However, they can also affect normal cells that divide rapidly, such as those in the bone marrow, digestive tract, and hair follicles, which can lead to side effects.

Chemotherapy can be given in a variety of ways, including intravenously (through a vein), orally (in pill form), or topically (applied to the skin). The drugs may be given in cycles, with a period of treatment followed by a period of rest, to allow the body to recover.

The benefits of chemotherapy depend on the type and stage of cancer being treated, as well as the individual patient's response to the drugs. In some cases, chemotherapy can cure cancer, especially when used in combination with other treatments such as surgery or radiation therapy. In other cases, chemotherapy may be used to slow the growth of cancer, relieve symptoms, or prolong life.

Despite its effectiveness, chemotherapy can have side effects, which can vary depending on the drugs used, the dose, and the patient's overall health. Common side effects of chemotherapy include fatigue, nausea and vomiting, hair loss, and increased risk of infection. However, many side effects can be managed with medication or other treatments.

Overall, chemotherapy is a powerful tool in the fight against cancer, and its continued development and refinement has led to improved outcomes and quality of life for many cancer patients.

Commonly Used Chemotherapy Drugs Approved by the FDA

Here is a table of commonly used chemotherapy drugs approved by the FDA, their mechanism of action, and length of a treatment cycle:

Chemotherapy Drug	Mechanism of Action	Length of Treatment Cycle
Carboplatin	Alkylating agent, damages DNA	21-28 days
Cisplatin	Alkylating agent, damages DNA	21-28 days
Cyclophosphamide	Alkylating agent, damages DNA	21-28 days
Docetaxel	Microtubule inhibitor, prevents cell division	21-28 days
Doxorubicin	Anthracycline, damages DNA	21-28 days
Fluorouracil (5-FU)	Antimetabolite, inhibits DNA and RNA synthesis	Continuous infusion or 5 days every 28 days
Gemcitabine	Nucleoside analog, inhibits DNA synthesis	21-28 days

	Microtubule inhibitor, prevents cell division	Weekly or every 21-28 days
Paclitaxel	Microtubule inhibitor, prevents cell division	Weekly or every 21-28 days
Vinblastine	Microtubule inhibitor, prevents cell division	Weekly or every 21-28 days
Vincristine	Microtubule inhibitor, prevents cell division	Weekly or every 21-28 days

Let's look at a cancer patient success story with chemotherapy: Lisa Newton was diagnosed with Stage III breast cancer at age 48 in January 2019, after finding a lump in her breast during a self-exam. Her doctor recommended a treatment plan that included chemotherapy, followed by surgery and radiation.

Lisa began chemotherapy in February 2019, which consisted of a combination of the drugs doxorubicin and cyclophosphamide, followed by paclitaxel. She received her treatment every two weeks over the course of several months. During her treatment, Lisa experienced some side effects such as nausea, fatigue, and hair loss, but her medical team helped her manage these symptoms with medication and other strategies. After completing her chemotherapy, Lisa underwent surgery to remove the tumor and nearby lymph nodes. The surgery was successful, and Lisa's medical team determined that she did not need radiation therapy.

Today, Lisa is cancer-free and continues to receive regular check-ups with her medical team to ensure that her cancer does not return.

Here is a table showing how chemotherapy is used in the treatment, whether early stage or advanced stage, of lung cancer, breast cancer, colon cancer, prostate cancer, and pancreatic cancer:

Cancer Type	Early Stage Treatment	Advanced Stage Treatment
Lung Cancer	Adjuvant chemotherapy following surgery	Chemotherapy may be used as the primary treatment for stage III or IV lung cancer, or in combination with radiation therapy
Breast Cancer	Adjuvant chemotherapy following surgery	Chemotherapy is often used in combination with targeted therapy for advanced stage breast cancer that has spread beyond the breast and nearby lymph nodes
Colon Cancer	Adjuvant chemotherapy following surgery	Chemotherapy may be used as the primary treatment for advanced colon cancer, or in combination with surgery and radiation therapy
Prostate Cancer	Not typically used in early stage	Chemotherapy may be used in combination with hormone therapy for advanced prostate cancer that is hormone-resistant and/or has spread beyond the prostate gland
Pancreatic Cancer	Not typically used in early stage	Chemotherapy may be used as the primary treatment for advanced pancreatic cancer, in combination with radiation therapy; chemotherapy may also be used following

		surgery to reduce the risk of cancer recurrence

A) Lung Cancer Chemotherapy

Here is a table showing the most commonly used chemotherapy drugs for lung cancer treatment, their percentage of procedures, and a brief description of each option:

Chemotherapy Drug	Percentage of Procedures	Description
Cisplatin	30%	Cisplatin is a platinum-containing chemotherapy drug that works by interfering with the DNA in cancer cells, preventing them from dividing and growing. It is typically used in combination with other chemotherapy drugs to treat advanced non-small cell lung cancer.
Carboplatin	25%	Carboplatin is also a platinum-containing chemotherapy drug that works similarly to cisplatin, but is generally less toxic. It is used in combination with other chemotherapy drugs to treat both small cell and non-small cell lung cancer.
Paclitaxel	20%	Paclitaxel is a taxane chemotherapy drug that

Drug	Percentage	Description
		works by preventing cancer cells from dividing and growing. It is typically used in combination with other chemotherapy drugs to treat advanced non-small cell lung cancer.
Gemcitabine	15%	Gemcitabine is a nucleoside analog chemotherapy drug that works by interfering with the DNA in cancer cells, preventing them from dividing and growing. It is often used in combination with other chemotherapy drugs to treat advanced non-small cell lung cancer.
Vinorelbine	10%	Vinorelbine is a vinca alkaloid chemotherapy drug that works by preventing cancer cells from dividing and growing. It is often used in combination with other chemotherapy drugs to treat advanced non-small cell lung cancer.

B) Breast Cancer Chemotherapy

here is a table showing the most commonly used chemotherapy drugs for breast cancer treatment, their percentage of procedures, and a brief description of each option:

Chemotherapy Drug	Percentage of Procedures	Brief Description
Doxorubicin (Adriamycin)	22.2%	An anthracycline chemotherapy drug that is effective against breast cancer. It works by interfering with the DNA in cancer cells and preventing them from dividing and growing.
Cyclophosphamide (Cytoxan)	22.0%	A chemotherapy drug that is often used in combination with other drugs to treat breast cancer. It works by interfering with the DNA in cancer cells and preventing them from dividing and growing.
Paclitaxel (Taxol)	20.4%	A chemotherapy drug that is used to treat breast cancer that has spread beyond the breast. It works by preventing cancer cells from dividing and growing by disrupting the normal function of microtubules.
Docetaxel (Taxotere)	12.5%	A chemotherapy drug that is used to treat breast cancer that has spread beyond the breast. It works by preventing cancer cells from dividing and growing by disrupting the normal function of microtubules.
Fluorouracil (5-FU)	7.6%	A chemotherapy drug that is used in combination with other drugs to treat breast cancer. It works by interfering with the DNA in cancer cells and preventing them from dividing and growing.

C) Colon Cancer Chemotherapy

Here is a table showing the most commonly used chemotherapy drugs for colon cancer treatment, their percentage of procedures, and a brief description of each option:

Chemotherapy drug	Percentage of procedures	Description
Fluorouracil (5-FU)	40-50%	5-FU is a type of antimetabolite chemotherapy drug that interferes with the metabolism of cancer cells. It is often used in combination with other chemotherapy drugs to treat colon cancer.
Capecitabine (Xeloda)	20-30%	Capecitabine is an oral chemotherapy drug that is converted into 5-FU in the body. It is often used as an alternative to 5-FU in the treatment of colon cancer.
Oxaliplatin (Eloxatin)	20-30%	Oxaliplatin is a type of platinum-based chemotherapy drug that interferes with the DNA in cancer cells, preventing them from dividing and growing. It is often used in combination with 5-FU or capecitabine to treat advanced colon cancer.
Irinotecan (Camptosar)	10-20%	Irinotecan is a type of topoisomerase inhibitor chemotherapy drug that interferes with the enzymes involved in DNA replication. It is often used in combination

	with 5-FU or capecitabine to treat advanced colon cancer.

D) Prostate Cancer Chemotherapy

Here is a table showing the most commonly used chemotherapy drugs for prostate cancer treatment, their percentage of procedures, and a brief description of each option:

Chemotherapy Drug	Percentage of Procedures	Description
Docetaxel (Taxotere)	40%	Taxotere is a type of taxane chemotherapy drug that works by preventing cancer cells from dividing and growing. It is administered intravenously every three weeks and is used to treat advanced prostate cancer that has spread to other parts of the body.
Cabazitaxel (Jevtana)	30%	Jevtana is also a type of taxane chemotherapy drug that works similarly to Taxotere. It is administered intravenously every three weeks and is used to treat advanced prostate cancer that has already been treated with other chemotherapy drugs, such as Taxotere.
Mitoxantrone (Novantrone)	20%	Novantrone is a chemotherapy drug that works by damaging the DNA of cancer cells and preventing them from dividing and growing. It is administered intravenously every three weeks and is used to treat advanced prostate cancer that has

		spread to other parts of the body and is no longer responding to hormone therapy.

E) Pancreatic Cancer Chemotherapy

Here's a table showing some of the most commonly used chemotherapy drugs for pancreatic cancer treatment, their percentage of use, and a brief description of each option:

Chemotherapy Drug	Percentage of Use	Description
Gemcitabine	>50%	Gemcitabine is a standard chemotherapy drug used to treat pancreatic cancer. It is given by injection into a vein and works by interfering with the growth and spread of cancer cells.
FOLFIRINOX	~25%	FOLFIRINOX is a combination chemotherapy regimen that includes four drugs: 5-fluorouracil, leucovorin, irinotecan, and oxaliplatin. It is used to treat advanced pancreatic cancer and has been shown to improve survival compared to gemcitabine alone.
Abraxane (Nab-paclitaxel)	~10%	Abraxane is a chemotherapy drug that is used in combination with gemcitabine to treat pancreatic cancer. It is given by injection into a vein and works by interfering with the growth and spread of

Drug		Description
		cancer cells. It is a newer drug that has shown promising results in clinical trials.
5-Fluorouracil (5-FU)	<10%	5-FU is a chemotherapy drug that is used to treat pancreatic cancer, often in combination with other drugs. It is given by injection into a vein and works by interfering with the growth and spread of cancer cells.
Cisplatin	<10%	Cisplatin is a chemotherapy drug that is used to treat pancreatic cancer, often in combination with other drugs. It is given by injection into a vein and works by interfering with the growth and spread of cancer cells.

To manage the side effects of chemotherapy, doctors use a variety of techniques. One of the most important is to tailor the chemotherapy regimen to the patient's individual needs, taking into account factors such as age, overall health, and the type and stage of cancer. Doctors also use medications to help manage side effects, such as anti-nausea drugs to help with nausea and vomiting, and pain medications to help with pain. In addition, patients may be advised to make lifestyle changes such as eating a healthy diet, staying hydrated, and getting regular exercise to help manage side effects.

While traditional chemotherapy can be an effective cancer treatment, it can also cause side effects due to the fact that the drugs used to treat cancer can also damage normal cells in the body. Recent advances in chemotherapy have focused on improving the effectiveness of the drugs while reducing the severity of side effects.

One of the recent advances in chemotherapy is the development of targeted therapy drugs, which are designed to attack specific cancer cells with minimal damage to normal cells and we will get into more details in later chapters. Targeted therapy drugs work by targeting specific molecules on cancer cells that are involved in their growth and survival, making them a more precise and effective way to treat cancer. Examples of targeted therapy drugs include trastuzumab (Herceptin) for breast cancer, bevacizumab (Avastin) for colorectal cancer, and imatinib (Gleevec) for chronic myeloid leukemia.

Another advance in chemotherapy is the development of immunotherapy drugs, which help the immune system to recognize and destroy cancer cells, and we will also get into more details in later chapters. Immunotherapy drugs work by blocking proteins on cancer cells that prevent the immune system from recognizing them as foreign, or by boosting the immune system's ability to attack cancer cells. Examples of immunotherapy drugs include pembrolizumab (Keytruda) and nivolumab (Opdivo) for lung cancer and melanoma.

More details on targeted therapy and immunotherapy are covered in the next two chapters.

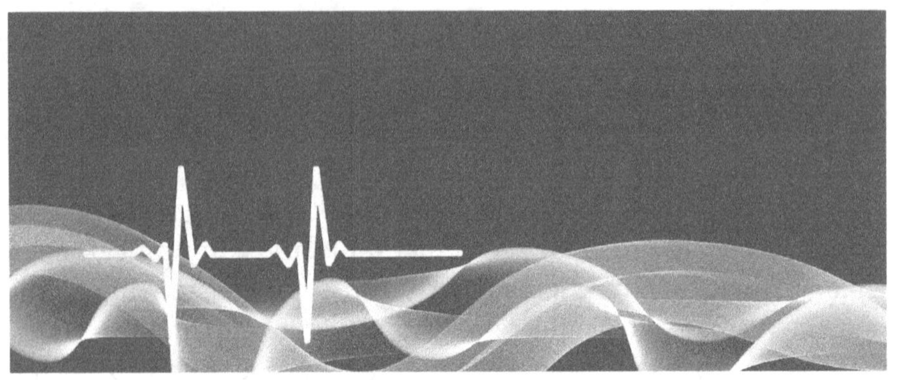

CHAPTER 7 TARGETED THERAPY
AS A CANCER TREATMENT OPTION

Targeted therapy is a type of cancer treatment that uses drugs to target specific molecules involved in the growth and spread of cancer cells. It was developed in the late 1990s and early 2000s as a result of advancements in the understanding of the biology of cancer cells and the identification of specific molecular targets.

The basic principle of targeted therapy is to identify specific proteins, enzymes, or other molecules that are involved in the development and growth of cancer cells and then use drugs to interfere with these targets. The drugs used in targeted therapy are designed to selectively bind to these specific targets, which can be located on the surface of cancer cells or inside them. Once the drug binds to the target, it can block the activity of the molecule and prevent the cancer cells from growing and dividing.

Targeted therapy has several benefits over traditional chemotherapy. Because the drugs are designed to specifically target cancer cells, they are less likely to damage healthy cells and cause side effects. This means that patients may experience fewer side effects, such as hair loss and nausea, than they would with conventional chemotherapy. Additionally, targeted therapy can be more effective than chemotherapy in certain types of cancer because it is tailored to the specific molecular characteristics of the cancer cells.

There are several different types of targeted therapy drugs, including monoclonal antibodies, tyrosine kinase inhibitors, and proteasome inhibitors. Monoclonal antibodies are designed to target specific proteins on the surface of cancer cells and can be used to stimulate the immune system to attack the cancer cells or to block the activity of proteins that are promoting the growth of cancer cells. Tyrosine kinase inhibitors work by blocking the activity of enzymes that are involved in cell signaling pathways that promote cancer cell growth. Proteasome inhibitors interfere with the breakdown of proteins in cancer cells, leading to cell death.

Targeted therapy has been approved for use in the treatment of several different types of cancer, including breast cancer, lung cancer, colorectal cancer, and leukemia, among others. However, targeted therapy is not effective for all types of cancer, and not all patients will respond to targeted therapy. It is important to discuss the risks and benefits of targeted therapy with a healthcare provider to determine if it is a suitable treatment option.

To determine if a targeted therapy is suitable for a cancer patient, several tests may be performed. These tests may include:

1. Biomarker testing: This involves analyzing a tumor tissue sample for specific genetic or protein mutations that are known to be targets for certain drugs.

2. Immunohistochemistry (IHC): This test involves using antibodies to detect specific proteins on the surface of cancer cells, which can help identify the type of cancer and potential

treatment options.

3. Polymerase chain reaction (PCR): This is a molecular biology technique used to amplify specific genes or sequences, which can help identify mutations in the DNA of cancer cells.

4. Next-generation sequencing (NGS): This is a genetic test that can detect mutations in multiple genes simultaneously, providing a comprehensive analysis of a patient's tumor.

5. Liquid biopsy: This involves analyzing a patient's blood for circulating tumor cells or fragments of DNA shed by tumor cells, which can help identify mutations that may be targeted by certain drugs.

These tests can help determine if a patient is a candidate for targeted therapy and which drugs may be most effective in treating their specific type of cancer.

Here is a table of some of the most commonly used targeted therapy drugs approved by the FDA for blood cancers, their mechanisms of action, and treatment cycle lengths:

Targeted Therapy Drug	Type of Blood Cancer Treated	Mechanism of Action	Length of Treatment Cycle
Imatinib (Gleevec)	Chronic myeloid leukemia	Inhibits BCR-ABL tyrosine kinase	Long-term, can be indefinite
Rituximab (Rituxan)	Non-Hodgkin lymphoma	Targets CD20 protein on B-cells	Varies, typically several months
Ibrutinib (Imbruvica)	Chronic lymphocytic leukemia, mantle cell lymphoma	Inhibits Bruton's tyrosine kinase	Long-term, can be indefinite
Venetoclax (Venclexta)	Chronic lymphocytic leukemia, acute myeloid leukemia	Inhibits B-cell lymphoma 2 (BCL-2) protein	Varies, typically several months
Brentuximab vedotin (Adcetris)	Hodgkin lymphoma, systemic anaplastic large cell lymphoma	Targets CD30 protein on lymphoma cells	Varies, typically several months
Blinatumomab (Blincyto)	Acute lymphoblastic leukemia	Bispecific T-cell engager (BiTE) that targets	Varies, typically several months

	CD19 protein on leukemia cells and CD3 protein on T-cells

Here is a table of commonly used FDA-approved targeted therapy drugs for solid cancers:

Targeted Therapy Drug	Type of Cancer Treated	Mechanism of Action	Length of Treatment Cycle
Trastuzumab (Herceptin)	Breast cancer	Targets HER2 protein to inhibit cell growth and division	Varies, can be given weekly or every three weeks
Lapatinib (Tykerb)	Breast cancer	Targets HER2 and EGFR proteins to inhibit cell growth and division	Varies, usually taken daily
Pertuzumab (Perjeta)	Breast cancer	Targets HER2 protein to inhibit cell growth and division	Varies, usually given every three weeks
Osimertinib (Tagrisso)	Lung Cancer	Targets EGFR protein to inhibit cell growth and division	Varies, usually taken daily
Bevacizumab (Avastin)	Colorectal, lung, kidney, ovarian, and cervical cancer	Inhibits angiogenesis (formation of new blood vessels) to prevent tumor growth	Varies, usually given every two or three weeks
Cetuximab (Erbitux)	Colorectal and head and neck cancer	Targets EGFR protein to inhibit cell growth and division	Varies, usually given weekly
Panitumumab (Vectibix)	Colorectal cancer	Targets EGFR protein to inhibit cell growth and division	Varies, usually given every two weeks
Sorafenib (Nexavar)	Liver, kidney, and thyroid cancer	Targets multiple signaling pathways to inhibit tumor growth and angiogenesis	Varies, taken twice daily
Sunitinib (Sutent)	Kidney and gastrointestinal stromal tumors	Targets multiple signaling pathways to inhibit tumor growth and angiogenesis	Varies, usually taken four weeks on and two weeks off
Imatinib (Gleevec)	Chronic myeloid leukemia, gastrointestinal stromal tumors	Targets abnormal protein produced by cancer cells to inhibit cell division	Varies, usually taken daily
Erlotinib (Tarceva)	Lung and pancreatic cancer	Targets EGFR protein to inhibit cell growth and division	Varies, usually taken daily
Crizotinib (Xalkori)	Non-small cell lung cancer	Targets ALK and ROS1 proteins to inhibit cell growth and division	Varies, usually taken twice daily
Olaparib (Lynparza)	Ovarian, breast, and pancreatic cancer	Targets PARP enzyme to prevent DNA repair in	Varies, usually taken twice daily

		cancer cells	
Pembrolizumab (Keytruda)	Multiple solid tumors (e.g. lung, melanoma, head and neck, bladder, etc.)	Targets PD-1 protein to enhance immune response against cancer cells	Varies, usually given every three weeks

Let's look at a cancer patient's success story with targeted therapy: John Doe was diagnosed with NSCLC in its early stages. Genetic testing revealed that his cancer had a mutation in the EGFR gene, making him a good candidate for targeted therapy with osimertinib. John started treatment with osimertinib and within a few weeks, he noticed a significant improvement in his symptoms. His cancerous tumors started to shrink and he was able to breathe better. John continued the treatment for several months, and follow-up scans showed that the tumors had continued to shrink. He was able to resume his normal activities and maintain a good quality of life. Targeted therapy with osimertinib had a significant impact on John's lung cancer and improved his overall prognosis.

A) Lung Cancer Targeted Therapy

Here is a table showing the most commonly used targeted therapy drugs for lung cancer treatment, their brand name, their percentage of procedures, and a brief description of each option:

Targeted Therapy Drug	Brand Name	Mechanism of Action	Percentage of Procedures
Osimertinib	Tagrisso	Inhibits EGFR T790M mutation	44%
Pembrolizumab	Keytruda	Inhibits PD-1 protein on T-cells	22%
Alectinib	Alecensa	Inhibits ALK gene rearrangement	14%

Crizotinib	Xalkori	Inhibits ALK gene rearrangement and ROS1 gene mutation	12%
Erlotinib	Tarceva	Inhibits EGFR mutation	4%
Brigatinib	Alunbrig	Inhibits ALK gene rearrangement	3%
Afatinib	Gilotrif	Inhibits EGFR mutation	1%

B) Breast Cancer Targeted Therapy

Here is a table showing the most commonly used targeted therapy drugs for breast cancer treatment, their brand name, mechanism of action, and their percentage of procedures

Targeted Therapy Drug	Brand Name	Mechanism of Action	Percentage of Procedures
Trastuzumab	Herceptin	Targets HER2 protein	20-25%
Pertuzumab	Perjeta	Targets HER2 protein	10-15%
Ado-trastuzumab emtansine	Kadcyla	Targets HER2 protein	5-10%
Palbociclib	Ibrance	Targets CDK4/6	15-20%
Ribociclib	Kisqali	Targets CDK4/6	5-10%
Abemaciclib	Verzenio	Targets CDK4/6	5-10%
Everolimus	Afinitor	Targets mTOR	5-10%
Fulvestrant	Faslodex	Targets estrogen	5-10%

C) Colon Cancer Targeted Therapy

Here is a table showing the most commonly used targeted therapy drugs for colon cancer treatment, their brand name, mechanism of action, and their percentage of procedures

Targeted Therapy Drug	Brand Name	Mechanism of Action	Percentage of Procedures
Bevacizumab	Avastin	Targets VEGF	28%
Cetuximab	Erbitux	Targets EGFR	10%
Panitumumab	Vectibix	Targets EGFR	8%
Regorafenib	Stivarga	Targets multiple kinases	3%
Trifluridine/Tipiracil	Lonsurf	Targets thymidine phosphorylase	2%

D) Prostate Cancer Targeted Therapy

Here is a table showing the most commonly used targeted therapy drugs for prostate cancer treatment, their brand name, mechanism of action, and their percentage of procedures:

Targeted Therapy Drug	Brand Name	Mechanism of Action	Percentage of Procedures
Enzalutamide	Xtandi	Androgen Receptor Inhibitor	50%
Abiraterone acetate	Zytiga	Androgen Synthesis Inhibitor	30%
Apalutamide	Erleada	Androgen Receptor Inhibitor	15%
Radium-223 dichloride	Xofigo	Alpha Particle Emitter	5%

E) Pancreatic Cancer Targeted Therapy

It's worth noting that pancreatic cancer is a challenging disease to treat, and targeted therapy options for it are relatively limited compared to other types of cancer. As a result, the use of chemotherapy and radiation therapy is more common in the treatment of pancreatic cancer. here's a table showing the most commonly used targeted therapy drugs for pancreatic cancer treatment, their brand name, mechanism of action, and their percentage of procedures:

Targeted Therapy Drug	Brand Name	Mechanism of Action	Percentage of Procedures
Erlotinib	Tarceva	Inhibits EGFR tyrosine kinase activity	19%
Bevacizumab	Avastin	Inhibits angiogenesis by binding to VEGF	13%
Gemcitabine + Abraxane	---	Gemcitabine: inhibits DNA synthesis Abraxane: inhibits microtubule function	8%
Olaparib	Lynparza	Inhibits PARP enzyme involved in DNA repair	5%
Pembrolizumab	Keytruda	Inhibits PD-1 receptor on T cells	4%

Targeted therapy drugs can be associated with several side effects, which can vary based on the specific drug used and the patient's individual health status. The side effects can range from mild to severe and may include gastrointestinal symptoms, skin rashes, fatigue, and changes in blood counts. In some cases, targeted therapy drugs can also affect the liver, kidneys, or heart.

To manage the side effects of targeted therapy, healthcare providers typically use a multi-disciplinary approach that involves close monitoring of the patient's symptoms, supportive care interventions, and adjustments to the treatment regimen as needed. Some common strategies for managing side effects of targeted therapy include:

1. Monitoring: Regular monitoring of the patient's vital signs, blood counts, and organ function can help healthcare providers identify any potential side effects early on.

2. Medications: Several medications, such as anti-diarrheal agents, anti-nausea drugs, and pain relievers, can be used to manage specific side effects of targeted therapy drugs.

3. Supportive care: Nutritional support, hydration, and rest can help patients manage fatigue and other symptoms associated with targeted therapy.

4. Dose adjustments: In some cases, healthcare providers may need to adjust the dose or schedule of targeted therapy drugs to minimize side effects while still providing effective treatment.

5. Patient education: Patients receiving targeted therapy should be educated about the potential side effects of their treatment, as well as strategies for managing them. This can help patients feel more in control of their treatment and better equipped to cope with any adverse effects that may occur.

In recent years, there have been additional advances in targeted therapy for cancer treatment, including the development of new drugs that target specific genetic mutations or pathways involved in tumor growth. This personalized approach to cancer treatment has shown promising results in clinical trials and is expected to play an increasingly important role in cancer care in the years to come. Additionally, researchers are exploring new methods for delivering targeted therapy, such as nanoparticles and gene therapy, which could potentially enhance the efficacy of these treatments while minimizing side effects.

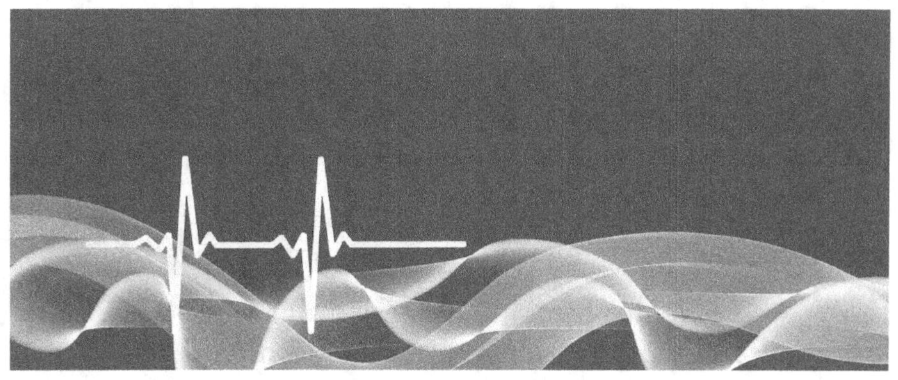

CHAPTER 8 IMMUNOTHERAPY AS A CANCER TREATMENT OPTION

Immunotherapy is a type of cancer treatment that uses the body's own immune system to fight cancer. It works by using substances made either by the body or in a laboratory to boost or restore the immune system's ability to recognize and destroy cancer cells.

The idea of using the immune system to fight cancer dates back to the late 19th century, when doctors observed that some cancer patients experienced spontaneous remissions of their disease following an infection. This suggested that the immune system was playing a role in controlling cancer.

In the 20th century, the development of more sophisticated tools and techniques allowed researchers to begin exploring the use of immunotherapy in a more targeted way. The discovery of immune checkpoint molecules such as CTLA-4 and PD-1 led to the development of drugs that block these molecules, enabling T cells to attack cancer cells more effectively. These drugs, known as immune checkpoint inhibitors, have revolutionized cancer treatment in recent years.

Immunotherapy can work in several ways, depending on the

specific type of treatment. Some types of immunotherapy work by boosting the immune system's overall ability to recognize and attack cancer cells. Others work by targeting specific molecules on the surface of cancer cells, making them more visible to the immune system.

There are several different types of immunotherapies, including:

1. Checkpoint inhibitors: These drugs work by blocking certain proteins on cancer cells or immune cells, which can help the immune system recognize and attack cancer cells.

2. CAR-T cell therapy: This type of immunotherapy involves genetically modifying a patient's T cells, a type of immune cell, to recognize and attack cancer cells.

3. Cancer vaccines: These vaccines work by stimulating the immune system to recognize and attack cancer cells.

4. Immune system modulators: These drugs work by stimulating the immune system to recognize and attack cancer cells.

PD-1 inhibitors block the interaction between the programmed cell death protein 1 (PD-1) receptor on T-cells and PD-1 ligands on cancer cells, thus enhancing the immune response against cancer. CTLA-4 inhibitors block the interaction between the cytotoxic T-lymphocyte-associated protein 4 (CTLA-4) receptor on T-cells and B7 ligands on cancer cells, which also enhances the immune response against cancer. PD-L1 inhibitors block the interaction between the programmed death-ligand 1 (PD-L1) on cancer cells and PD-1 receptors on T-cells, thus preventing cancer cells from evading the immune response.

CAR T-cell therapy involves the collection of a patient's T-cells, which are genetically modified to express chimeric antigen receptors (CARs) specific for a cancer cell surface antigen. The CAR T-cells are then infused back into the patient, where they target and destroy cancer cells expressing the antigen.

The benefits of immunotherapy include:

1. Targeted treatment: Immunotherapy can be targeted to specific types of cancer cells, reducing the risk of damage to healthy cells.

2. Long-term effects: Immunotherapy can continue to work even after treatment has ended, providing long-term benefits, because the immune system has a "memory" of past infections and cancer cells.

3. Fewer side effects: Compared to traditional cancer treatments such as chemotherapy and radiation therapy, immunotherapy often has fewer side effects.

4. Personalized treatment: Immunotherapy can be tailored to each patient's individual needs, based on their specific type of cancer and other factors.

Additionally, because immunotherapy works by harnessing the body's own immune system, it has the potential to be effective against a wide range of cancers, including those that are difficult to treat with traditional therapies.

Several tests may be performed to determine if immunotherapy is suitable for a cancer patient, including:

1. Tumor biomarker testing: Biomarker testing is used to identify specific proteins, genetic mutations, or other markers present on or within cancer cells that can be targeted by immunotherapy drugs.

2. Genetic testing: Genetic testing is performed to identify specific mutations or genetic alterations that may be targeted by certain types of immunotherapy drugs.

3. PD-L1 testing: PD-L1 testing is used to measure the levels of

PD-L1, a protein that is often overexpressed on the surface of cancer cells and is used to determine the potential benefit of PD-1 or PD-L1 inhibitors.

4. Tumor mutational burden (TMB) testing: TMB testing is used to identify the number of mutations present in a tumor, which can help determine the potential effectiveness of immunotherapy drugs that target specific mutations.

5. Microsatellite instability (MSI) testing: MSI testing is used to determine whether a tumor has a high level of genetic instability, which may indicate that it will respond well to immunotherapy.

The specific tests used may vary depending on the type of cancer and the type of immunotherapy being considered.

Commonly Used Immunotherapy Drugs Approved by the FDA

Here is a table of commonly used immunotherapy drugs approved by the FDA, their mechanism of action, and the length of a treatment cycle:

Drug name	Mechanism of action	Length of treatment cycle
Pembrolizumab (Keytruda)	PD-1 inhibitor	Every 3-6 weeks
Nivolumab (Opdivo)	PD-1 inhibitor	Every 2 weeks
Ipilimumab (Yervoy)	CTLA-4 inhibitor	Every 3-4 weeks
Atezolizumab (Tecentriq)	PD-L1 inhibitor	Every 2-3 weeks
Durvalumab (Imfinzi)	PD-L1 inhibitor	Every 4 weeks
Avelumab (Bavencio)	PD-L1 inhibitor	Every 2 weeks
Tisagenlecleucel (Kymriah)	CAR T-cell therapy	Single infusion
Axicabtagene ciloleucel (Yescarta)	CAR T-cell therapy	Single infusion

The length of a treatment cycle for these drugs varies depending on the specific drug and the type of cancer being treated.

Let's look at a cancer patient's success story with immunotherapy: Melinda Bachini was diagnosed with stage IV metastatic melanoma in 2014, which had spread to her lungs, liver, and spine. She underwent several rounds of chemotherapy and radiation, but her tumors continued to grow. Her doctors then suggested she try a newer form of treatment: immunotherapy.

Melinda began receiving a drug called pembrolizumab, which is an immune checkpoint inhibitor that blocks a protein called PD-1, allowing the immune system to attack cancer cells. After just four rounds of treatment, Melinda's tumors had shrunk significantly. She continued on the drug, and after a year of treatment, her scans showed no evidence of cancer.

Melinda's success with immunotherapy led to her becoming an advocate for the treatment, and she even had the opportunity to meet with former Vice President Joe Biden to discuss the importance of cancer research funding.

A) Lung Cancer Immunotherapy

Here is a table showing the most commonly used immunotherapy drugs for lung cancer treatment, their percentage of procedures, and a brief description of each option:

Immunotherapy Drug	Percentage of Procedures	Mechanism of Action
Pembrolizumab (Keytruda)	30%	Targets PD-1 protein to help the immune system recognize and destroy cancer cells.

Nivolumab (Opdivo)	25%	Targets PD-1 protein to help the immune system recognize and destroy cancer cells.
Atezolizumab (Tecentriq)	15%	Targets PD-L1 protein to help the immune system recognize and destroy cancer cells.
Durvalumab (Imfinzi)	10%	Targets PD-L1 protein to help the immune system recognize and destroy cancer cells.
Ipilimumab (Yervoy)	5%	Targets CTLA-4 protein to help the immune system recognize and destroy cancer cells.

Currently, there are no immunotherapy drugs approved by the FDA specifically for breast cancer treatment. However, some immunotherapy drugs are used in combination with chemotherapy for certain types of breast cancer, such as triple-negative breast cancer. These drugs include pembrolizumab and atezolizumab.

B)   Breast Cancer Immunotherapy

Here is a table showing the immunotherapy drugs used in combination with chemotherapy for triple-negative breast cancer:

Immunotherapy Drug	Brand Name	Mechanism of Action	Percentage of Procedures
Pembrolizumab	Keytruda	Targets PD-1 protein on immune cells to help identify and attack cancer cells	25-30%
Atezolizumab	Tecentriq	Blocks PD-L1 protein on cancer cells, allowing immune cells to attack them	40-50%

C) Colon Cancer Immunotherapy

here is a table showing the most commonly used immunotherapy drugs for colon cancer treatment, their percentage of procedures, and a brief description of each option

Drug name	Brand name	Percentage of procedures	Mechanism of action
Pembrolizumab	Keytruda	40%	Blocks PD-1 protein on T cells from binding to PD-L1 on cancer cells, allowing T cells to attack cancer cells
Nivolumab	Opdivo	20%	Blocks PD-1 protein on T cells from binding to PD-L1 on cancer cells, allowing T cells to attack cancer cells

			Blocks CTLA-4 protein on T cells from binding to cancer cells, allowing T cells to attack cancer
Ipilimumab	Yervoy	10%	cells
			Blocks PD-L1 protein on cancer cells, allowing T cells to attack cancer
Atezolizumab	Tecentriq	10%	cells
			Blocks PD-L1 protein on cancer cells, allowing T cells to attack cancer
Durvalumab	Imfinzi	10%	cells

D) Prostate Cancer Immunotherapy

Here's a table showing the most commonly used immunotherapy drugs for prostate cancer treatment, their brand name, their percentage of procedures, and a brief description of each option:

Immunotherapy Drug	Brand Name	Percentage of Procedures	Brief Description
Sipuleucel-T	Provenge	100%	A personalized immunotherapy that involves collecting a patient's white blood cells, exposing them to a protein found in most prostate cancers, and then re-infusing the cells back into the patient's body to stimulate an immune response against the cancer.
Pembrolizumab	Keytruda	<1%	A checkpoint inhibitor that

			blocks a protein called PD-1 on T cells, allowing them to attack cancer cells more effectively. Approved for use in advanced prostate cancer with specific genetic mutations.
Nivolumab	Opdivo	<1%	A checkpoint inhibitor that blocks a protein called PD-1 on T cells, allowing them to attack cancer cells more effectively. Approved for use in advanced prostate cancer with specific genetic mutations.
Ipilimumab	Yervoy	<1%	A checkpoint inhibitor that blocks a protein called CTLA-4 on T cells, allowing them to attack cancer cells more effectively. Approved for use in advanced prostate cancer with specific genetic mutations.

Note that Sipuleucel-T is currently the only FDA-approved immunotherapy for prostate cancer, and it has a unique mechanism of action compared to checkpoint inhibitors like Pembrolizumab, Nivolumab, and Ipilimumab. Checkpoint inhibitors may be used off-label for certain types of advanced prostate cancer with specific genetic mutations, but more research is needed to fully understand their efficacy in this context.

E)   Pancreatic Cancer Immunotherapy

Unfortunately, there are currently no FDA-approved immunotherapy drugs for the treatment of pancreatic cancer.

Like all cancer treatments, immunotherapy can cause side effects, but they are usually different from those caused by traditional chemotherapy or radiation therapy.

Side effects of immunotherapy can vary depending on the type of treatment and the specific drugs used, but some common side effects include fatigue, fever, chills, nausea and vomiting, diarrhea, skin rash, itching, high or low blood pressure, headaches, muscle or joint pain etc

Patients should report any side effects to their healthcare team as soon as possible so that they can be managed appropriately. In some cases, treatment may need to be stopped or the dose adjusted to manage the side effects.

Here are some strategies for managing common side effects of immunotherapy:

1. Fatigue: Get plenty of rest and avoid overexertion. Gentle exercise, such as walking or yoga, may also help.

2. Nausea and vomiting: Avoid strong smells, eat small meals frequently throughout the day, and stay hydrated.

3. Skin rash and itching: Keep the affected area clean and moisturized. Avoid scratching or rubbing the skin.

4. High or low blood pressure: Monitor your blood pressure regularly and follow your doctor's recommendations for managing it.

5. Headaches: Take over-the-counter pain relievers, such as acetaminophen, as directed by your doctor.

6. Muscle or joint pain: Gentle exercise and stretching, as well as over-the-counter pain relievers, can help manage this side effect.

Recent advances in immunotherapy include the development of new drugs and combinations of drugs, as well as new techniques for identifying patients who are most likely to benefit from immunotherapy. Some of the latest developments include:

1. Combination therapy: Researchers are exploring the use of combination immunotherapy treatments, which may be more effective than single-agent therapy. Combining different types of immunotherapies, such as checkpoint inhibitors and CAR T-cell therapy, may also enhance their effectiveness.

2. Cell-based immunotherapy: CAR T-cell therapy is one type of cell-based immunotherapy, but other types such as Tumor infiltrating lymphocytes (TIL) is also being developed.

3. Biomarker testing: Biomarker testing can help identify patients who are most likely to benefit from immunotherapy. For example, some immunotherapy drugs work best in patients whose tumors express certain biomarkers, such as PD-L1.

4. Development of new drugs: Researchers are continuing to develop new immunotherapy drugs and are exploring new targets for these drugs. For example, new drugs that target immune checkpoint molecules other than PD-1 and CTLA-4 are currently in development.

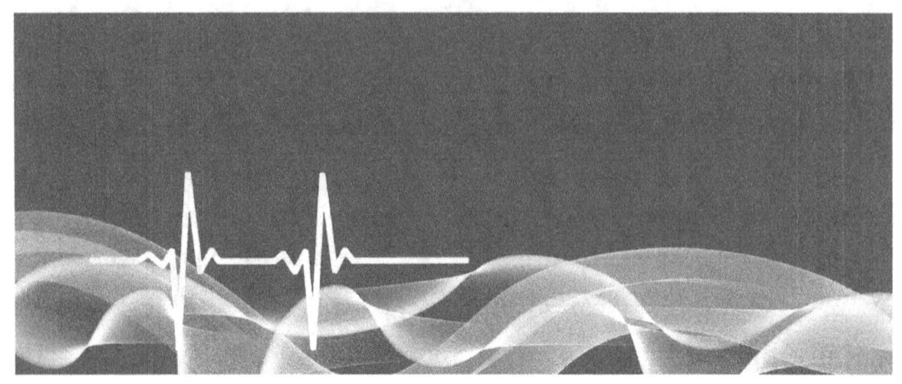

CHAPTER 9 INTEGRATIVE AND ALTERNATIVE TREATMENT ON CANCER AS AN OPTION

Integrative and alternative therapies (IAT) for cancer treatment is a broad term that encompasses a range of therapies and practices that fall outside of mainstream medicine, it can encompass a range of approaches that complement conventional cancer treatments such as chemotherapy, radiation therapy, and surgery. These approaches are sometimes used alongside conventional treatments to help manage symptoms and improve quality of life, while other times they may be used in lieu of conventional treatments. IAT can include a variety of interventions, such as nutritional and herbal supplements, acupuncture, massage therapy, meditation, and yoga.

The use of complementary and alternative medicine (CAM) dates back thousands of years. Traditional Chinese medicine, Ayurveda, and other ancient healing systems have long incorporated natural remedies and holistic approaches to treating illness including cancer. The use of complementary therapies alongside conventional cancer treatments gained popularity in the 1970s, with the founding of the American Holistic Medical Association. Today, IAT is becoming increasingly popular, and many cancer centers now offer integrative services alongside conventional treatments.

The use of IAT for cancer treatment is based on the idea that it can help support the body's natural healing mechanisms, improve the immune system's ability to fight cancer, and reduce the side effects of conventional cancer treatments. Many IAT approaches are aimed at improving overall health and well-being, with the belief that a healthy body is better able to fight cancer. Some IAT approaches may also directly target cancer cells, either by inhibiting their growth or promoting their destruction.

The benefits of IAT for cancer treatment can vary depending on the approach used. Some of the potential benefits include:

1. Reduced symptoms: IAT approaches such as acupuncture, massage therapy, and meditation can help reduce symptoms such as pain, anxiety, and fatigue.

2. Improved quality of life: Many IAT approaches are aimed at improving overall health and well-being, which can lead to a better quality of life for cancer patients.

3. Reduced side effects of conventional treatments: Some IAT approaches, such as acupuncture and nutritional supplements, may help reduce the side effects of chemotherapy and radiation therapy.

4. Improved immune function: Some IAT approaches, such as nutritional supplements and herbal remedies, may help improve immune function, which can aid in cancer treatment.

5. Enhanced sense of control: Many cancer patients feel a loss of control over their lives during treatment. IAT approaches such as meditation and yoga can help patients feel more in control and empowered.

It's important to note that while IAT may offer benefits for some cancer patients, it is not a substitute for conventional cancer treatment. It's essential that patients work closely with their healthcare team to develop an individualized treatment plan that incorporates both conventional and complementary therapies.

here's a table outlining some commonly used integrative and alternative therapies for cancer treatment, their mechanism of action, and the length of a treatment cycle.

Therapy	Mechanism of Action	Length of Treatment Cycle
Acupuncture	Stimulates the body's natural healing processes, reduces pain and inflammation	Usually administered in 6-12 weekly sessions
Herbal remedies	Contains natural compounds that may have anti-cancer properties, supports immune function	Taken over several weeks or months, under the guidance of a healthcare practitioner
Meditation	Reduces stress and anxiety, promotes relaxation and emotional balance	Usually practiced daily, with benefits seen after several weeks or months
Nutritional therapy	Provides the body with essential nutrients to support overall health and immune function	Ongoing, with adjustments made as needed based on individual response

Reiki	Balances the body's energy systems, promotes relaxation and emotional balance	Usually administered in 4-6 weekly sessions, with additional sessions as needed
Tai chi	Reduces stress and anxiety, promotes relaxation and physical balance	Usually practiced several times per week, with benefits seen after several weeks or months
Yoga	Reduces stress and anxiety, promotes relaxation and physical balance	Usually practiced several times per week, with benefits seen after several weeks or months

Here's a success story of a patient with breast cancer who incorporated integrative and alternative therapies into her treatment plan.

Patient: Cynthia B.

Condition: Breast cancer

Treatment: In addition to conventional cancer treatments such as chemotherapy and radiation therapy, Cynthia incorporated integrative and alternative therapies into her treatment plan. She worked with an integrative oncologist and a nutritionist at Memorial Sloan Kettering Cancer Center to develop a plan that included acupuncture, nutritional therapy, and mind-body therapies such as meditation and yoga.

Outcome: Cynthia found that incorporating these therapies into her treatment plan helped her manage the side effects of chemotherapy and radiation therapy. She also found that the mind-body therapies helped her cope with the emotional and psychological challenges of cancer. Cynthia is now cancer-free and continues to incorporate integrative and alternative therapies into her life as part of her overall wellness plan.

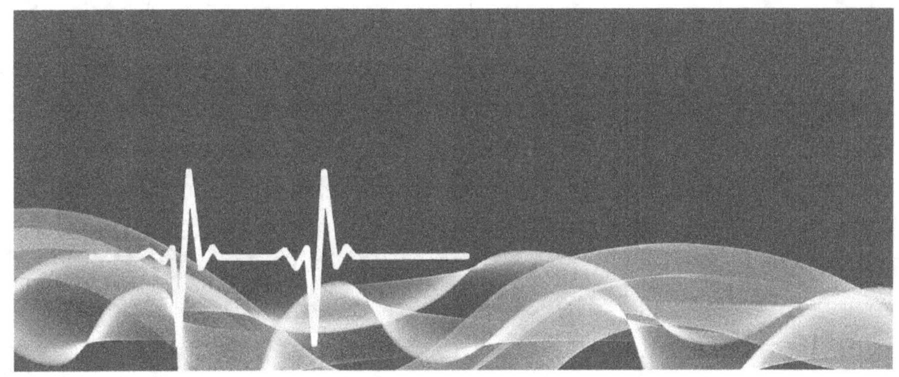

CHAPTER 10 FRONTIERS OF CANCER TREATMENT DEVELOPMENT

Research into new and innovative therapies is ongoing, and there are several promising approaches being explored in the field of oncology. The development of new treatments for cancers is essential to improve patient outcomes and reduce the cancer burden. Let's look at some frontiers of cancer treatment development, with a focus on lung cancer, breast cancer, colon cancer, prostate cancer, and pancreatic cancer.

New Approaches in Lung Cancer Treatment

Lung cancer is the leading cause of cancer-related deaths worldwide. It is a challenging disease to treat, with many patients presenting with advanced-stage disease at the time of diagnosis. However, recent advancements in immunotherapy have shown promising results in the treatment of lung cancer. Immunotherapy is a type of cancer treatment that works by stimulating the body's immune system to recognize and attack cancer cells.

One promising approach to immunotherapy is the use of cancer vaccines. Cancer vaccines work by training the immune system to recognize and attack cancer cells. There are currently several cancer vaccines in development for the treatment of lung cancer. For example, the TG4010 vaccine is a therapeutic vaccine that targets a protein called MUC1, which is overexpressed in many lung cancers. A phase II clinical trial of TG4010 showed promising results, with a median overall survival of 17.1 months in patients with advanced non-small cell lung cancer. Another example of a cancer vaccine for lung cancer is CIMAvax-EGF, which targets the epidermal growth factor (EGF) receptor on lung cancer cells. In clinical trials, CIMAvax-EGF has been shown to extend the lives of lung cancer patients.

Another promising approach to immunotherapy is the use of mRNA cancer vaccines. mRNA cancer vaccines work by delivering genetic material that instructs cells to produce proteins that stimulate the immune system to recognize and attack cancer cells. Moderna, a biotech company, has developed an mRNA cancer vaccine called mRNA-4157, which targets mutations commonly found in lung cancer. A phase I clinical trial of mRNA-4157 showed that the vaccine was safe and induced an immune response in patients with non-small cell lung cancer.

New Approaches in Breast Cancer Treatment

Breast cancer is the most diagnosed cancer in women worldwide. It is a heterogeneous disease, with different subtypes that have distinct biological characteristics and treatment responses. In recent years, there has been a growing interest in the use of adoptive T-cell therapy for the treatment of breast cancer. Adoptive T-cell therapy involves taking T-cells from a patient's own immune system, genetically modifying them to recognize and attack cancer cells, and then infusing them back into the patient.

One type of adoptive T-cell therapy that has shown promising results in the treatment of breast cancer is tumor-infiltrating lymphocyte (TIL) therapy. TIL therapy involves removing T-cells from a patient's tumor, expanding them in the laboratory, and then infusing them back into the patient. In a phase II clinical trial, TIL therapy resulted in a complete response in 20% of patients with metastatic triple-negative breast cancer, a subtype of breast cancer that is particularly challenging to treat.

Gene therapy involves the insertion of healthy genes into cancer cells to correct genetic mutations that cause cancer. One example of a gene therapy for breast cancer is the use of the p53 gene, which is often mutated in breast cancer cells. Researchers have developed a viral vector that can deliver the healthy p53 gene to breast cancer cells. In preclinical studies, this treatment has been shown to shrink breast tumors and improve survival rates.

Gene editing involves using CRISPR-Cas9 technology to target and edit specific genes in cancer cells. Researchers are exploring the use of gene editing to target the HER2 gene, which is overexpressed in some forms of breast cancer. By editing the HER2 gene, researchers hope to prevent the growth and spread of breast cancer cells.

New Approaches in Colon Cancer Treatment

Colon cancer is the third most commonly diagnosed cancer and the second leading cause of cancer-related deaths worldwide. Surgery is the primary treatment for early-stage colon cancer, while chemotherapy is typically used to treat advanced-stage disease. However, chemotherapy is associated with significant side effects, and there is a need for more targeted therapies.

Researchers are also exploring the use of TIL (tumor-infiltrating lymphocytes) therapy for colon cancer. TIL therapy involves removing T cells from a patient's tumor, growing them in the lab, and then infusing them back into the patient's body. The

T cells are trained to recognize and attack the patient's specific cancer cells. In a clinical trial of TIL therapy for colon cancer, patients who received the treatment had a higher rate of tumor shrinkage and longer progression-free survival compared to those who received standard chemotherapy.

One promising approach to the treatment of colon cancer is gene therapy. Gene therapy involves delivering genetic material to cancer cells to alter their behavior or kill them. Researchers have developed a gene therapy approach for colon cancer that involves delivering a virus that carries a gene called P53, which is commonly mutated in colon cancer. The P53 gene is a tumor suppressor gene that helps prevent cancer by regulating cell growth and division. In preclinical studies, the P53 gene therapy approach showed promising results in the treatment of colon cancer.

New Approaches in Prostate Cancer Treatment

Prostate cancer is the most common cancer in men. The primary treatment for localized prostate cancer is surgery or radiation therapy, while hormone therapy is typically used to treat advanced-stage disease. However, many patients develop resistance to hormone therapy over time, highlighting the need for new treatment approaches.

One emerging area of prostate cancer treatment is gene editing. Gene editing involves making precise changes to the DNA of cancer cells to alter their behavior or kill them. Researchers have developed a gene editing approach for prostate cancer that involves using CRISPR/Cas9 technology to target a gene called androgen receptor (AR), which is involved in the growth and progression of prostate cancer. In preclinical studies, the AR gene editing approach showed promising results in the treatment of prostate cancer.

Another promising technology is PSMA (prostate-specific

membrane antigen) PET imaging, which uses a radioactive tracer to detect PSMA on the surface of prostate cancer cells. PSMA PET imaging has been shown to be more accurate than traditional imaging techniques for detecting prostate cancer. This technology could help identify prostate cancer at an earlier stage and improve treatment outcomes.

New Approaches in Pancreatic Cancer Treatment

Pancreatic cancer is one of the deadliest forms of cancer, with a five-year survival rate of less than 10%. Surgery is the only curative treatment for pancreatic cancer, but many patients are not eligible for surgery due to the advanced stage of their disease. Chemotherapy is typically used to treat advanced-stage pancreatic cancer, but it is associated with significant side effects and only provides modest benefits.

One emerging area of pancreatic cancer treatment is the use of emerging imaging equipment. Pancreatic cancer is notoriously difficult to detect and treat due to its location deep within the abdomen. However, recent advancements in imaging technology, such as magnetic resonance imaging (MRI) and positron emission tomography (PET), are improving the detection and diagnosis of pancreatic cancer. These imaging techniques can provide high-resolution images of the pancreas and surrounding tissues, allowing for more accurate diagnosis and treatment planning.

Immunotherapy, gene therapy, gene editing, adoptive T-cell therapy, and emerging imaging equipment are all promising areas of cancer treatment development. While there is still much to learn about these approaches, the potential for improved cancer treatment outcomes is promising. With continued research and innovation, we can hope to see more success stories in the fight against cancer.

Resources for Latest Cancer Treatment Development

Here is a table about organizations, conferences and events

that follow the latest cancer treatment development and cancer clinical trial results.

Organization/Conference/Event	Brief Description	Website
National Comprehensive Cancer Network (NCCN)	The NCCN is a non-profit organization that provides guidelines for the treatment of various types of cancer. They also host an annual conference and provide resources for cancer care providers.	https://www.nccn.org/
American Association for Cancer Research (AACR)	The AACR is a professional organization for cancer researchers and physicians. They publish journals, host conferences, and provide funding for cancer research.	https://www.aacr.org/
American Society of Clinical Oncology (ASCO)	The ASCO is a professional organization for clinical oncologists. They host conferences and publish guidelines for cancer treatment.	https://www.asco.org/
European Society for Medical Oncology (ESMO)	The ESMO is a professional organization for medical oncologists in Europe. They host conferences and provide education and training for cancer professionals.	https://www.esmo.org/
Cancer Research UK	Cancer Research UK is a charity that funds cancer research and provides information about cancer. They also host events and fundraisers to support cancer research.	https://www.cancerresearchuk.org/
National Cancer Institute (NCI)	The NCI is a government agency that conducts and funds cancer research. They also provide information about cancer and support clinical trials.	https://www.cancer.gov/
World Cancer Congress	The World Cancer Congress is a conference hosted by the Union for International Cancer Control (UICC). It brings together cancer experts from around the world to share knowledge and discuss advances in cancer treatment.	https://www.worldcancercongress.org/

American Society of Hematology (ASH)	The ASH is a professional organization for hematologists. They host conferences and publish guidelines for the treatment of blood disorders, including some types of cancer.	https://www.hematology.org/
Society for Immunotherapy of Cancer (SITC)	The SITC is a professional organization for cancer immunotherapy researchers and physicians. They host conferences and provide education and training for cancer professionals.	https://www.sitcancer.org/
American Association of Cancer Institutes (AACI)	The AACI is a professional organization for cancer research institutions in the United States. They provide support and resources for cancer research and education.	https://www.aaci-cancer.org/
ClinicalTrials.gov	ClinicalTrials.gov is a database of clinical trials for cancer and other diseases. It provides information about ongoing and completed trials, including trial results.	https://clinicaltrials.gov/

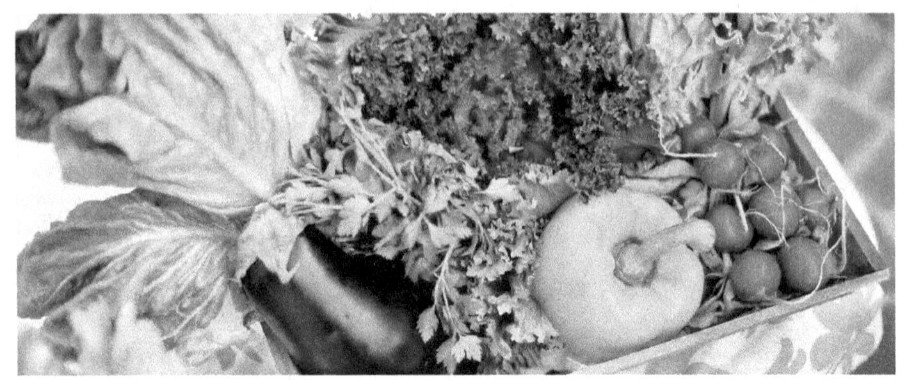

SECTION III CANCER PATIENT NUTRITION, DIET AND OFF-LABEL DRUG USE

Cancer treatments such as chemotherapy, radiation therapy, and surgery can take a toll on a patient's body. Proper nutrition is crucial for cancer patients as it helps support the immune system, reduce side effects, and improve overall quality of life. Nutrients can be divided into two categories: macronutrients and micronutrients. There are three macronutrients: carbohydrates, proteins, and fats. Carbohydrates are an important source of energy and should make up 45-65% of a cancer patient's daily caloric intake. Whole grains, fruits, and vegetables are good sources of complex carbohydrates that provide fiber, vitamins, and minerals. Proteins are essential for tissue repair and maintenance, and cancer patients should aim to consume 0.8-1.2 grams of protein per kilogram of body weight. Lean meats, fish, poultry, legumes, and dairy products are good sources of protein. Fat intake should be limited to 20-35% of daily caloric intake and should come from healthy sources such as olive oil, nuts, and avocados. On the other hand, micronutrients, such as vitamins and minerals, are essential for proper body function. Vitamin D, for example, is important for bone health and can be obtained from sunlight, fatty fish, and fortified dairy products. Calcium is also important for bone health and can be obtained from dairy products, leafy greens, and fortified foods. Cancer patients are usually deficient in micronutrients including Vitamin D and may also be at risk for deficiencies in vitamin B12 and folate, which can be found in animal products, fortified grains, and leafy greens. A diet rich in fruits and vegetables can provide cancer patients with important vitamins and minerals such as vitamin C, vitamin A, and potassium.

In this section, we will discuss the nutrition/diet considerations and strategies for cancer patients as well as off-label drug use.

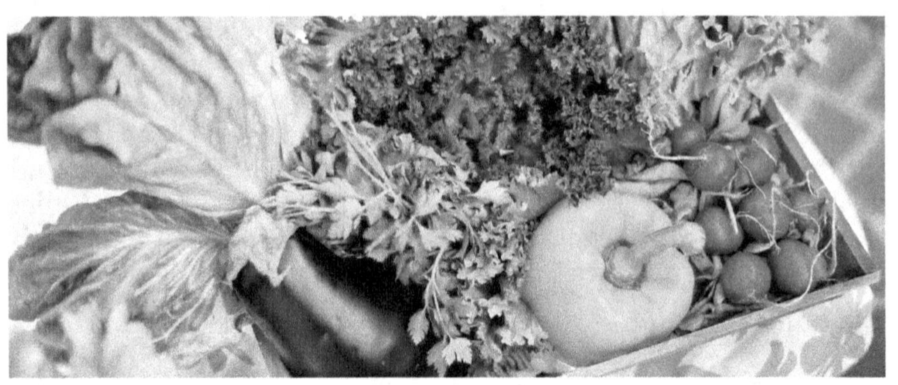

CHAPTER 11 KEY NUTRIENTS AND NUTRITION STRATEGIES FOR CANCER PATIENTS

Cancer treatments can often cause side effects such as nausea, vomiting, diarrhea, constipation, fatigue, and loss of appetite. These side effects can negatively impact a patient's ability to eat a healthy diet and maintain adequate nutrition, which is essential for recovery. Also, individual nutrition needs can vary a lot, therefore it is important for cancer patients to work closely with their healthcare team and a registered dietitian to develop a personalized nutrition plan that addresses their individual needs.

Key Nutrients for Cancer Patients

Below is a table showing key nutrients that are important for cancer patients and their food sources.

Nutrient	Examples of Food Sources
Protein	Lean meats, poultry, fish, eggs, beans, legumes

	Dairy products, tofu, tempeh, quinoa
Carbohydrates	Whole grains (brown rice, quinoa, whole wheat bread)
	Fruits, vegetables, legumes, beans
Healthy Fats	Avocados, nuts, seeds, olive oil, fatty fish
	Nut butter, flaxseed, chia seeds
Fiber	Whole grains, fruits, vegetables, legumes
	Nuts, seeds, bran cereals
Antioxidants	Berries (blueberries, strawberries, raspberries)
	Dark leafy greens, colorful fruits and vegetables
	Nuts, seeds, green tea, dark chocolate
Omega-3 Fatty Acids	Fatty fish (salmon, mackerel, sardines)
	Chia seeds, flaxseeds, walnuts
Vitamin D	Fatty fish, fortified dairy products, egg yolks
	Sunlight (limited exposure), supplements
Vitamin C	Citrus fruits (oranges, grapefruits, lemons)
	Bell peppers, strawberries, kiwi,

	broccoli
	Tomatoes, leafy greens
Zinc	Shellfish, lean meats, poultry, legumes
	Seeds, nuts, dairy products
Iron	Lean meats, poultry, fish, beans, legumes
	Fortified cereals, spinach, tofu
	Dried fruits (raisins, apricots)
Hydration	Water, herbal teas, broths, soups
	Fruits and vegetables with high water content
	Electrolyte drinks, low-sugar sports drink, homemade smoothies

In general, cancer patients need to consume enough calories to maintain their weight and energy levels, especially during treatment. However, many cancer treatments can cause a loss of appetite, which makes it challenging to consume enough calories. Therefore, it is important to focus on calorie-dense foods that provide a high number of calories in small portions. Examples include nuts, seeds, avocado, olive oil, cheese, and full-fat dairy products.

Cancer treatments can cause muscle wasting, which makes it difficult for patients to maintain their strength and mobility. Therefore, cancer patients need to consume enough protein to prevent muscle loss and promote recovery, as protein is crucial for cancer patients because it supports the growth and repair of cells and tissues. Examples of protein-rich foods include meat, poultry, fish, eggs, dairy products, legumes, nuts, and seeds.

Cancer treatments can also impact the body's ability to absorb essential vitamins and minerals, which can lead to deficiencies. Therefore, it is important for cancer patients to consume a variety of nutrient-dense foods that provide adequate amounts of vitamins and minerals. Examples include fruits, vegetables, whole grains, lean protein, dairy products, and healthy fats.

Cancer treatments can cause dehydration due to vomiting, diarrhea, and sweating, but proper hydration to stay hydrated is essential for cancer patients because it helps to flush toxins from the body, promotes healing, and supports normal body functions. Cancer patients should aim to drink plenty of fluids, e.g. at least eight glasses of water (64 oz) per day.

Nutrition Strategy for Cancer Patients: Dos and Don'ts

When working with a registered dietitian, it is useful for a cancer patient to follow specific strategies to come up with concrete and achievable plans. Here is a table outlining nutrition strategies for cancer patients, including dos and don'ts.

Nutrition Strategy	Dos	Don'ts
Balanced Diet	Include a variety of fruits, vegetables, whole grains, lean proteins, and healthy fats.	Avoid restrictive diets or extreme dietary changes without medical guidance.
Adequate Protein	Consume protein-rich foods like lean meats, poultry, fish, beans, legumes, dairy	Avoid excessive intake of processed meats or fried foods.

	products, and plant-based proteins.	
Hydration	Drink enough fluids to stay hydrated. Water, herbal teas, broths, and electrolyte drinks can help.	Avoid excessive intake of sugary beverages and alcohol.
Fiber	Include high-fiber foods like whole grains, fruits, vegetables, legumes, nuts, and seeds.	Avoid high-fiber foods if they cause discomfort or digestive issues.
Healthy Fats	Include sources of healthy fats such as avocados, nuts, seeds, olive oil, and fatty fish.	Limit consumption of saturated and trans fats found in processed and fried foods.
Antioxidant-Rich Foods	Consume foods rich in antioxidants like berries, dark leafy greens, colorful fruits, nuts, and green tea.	Avoid relying solely on antioxidant supplements without medical guidance.
Nutrient-Dense Foods	Choose nutrient-dense foods that provide a range of vitamins, minerals, and antioxidants.	Avoid empty calorie foods with limited nutritional value.
Small, Frequent Meals	Opt for smaller, more frequent meals to maintain energy	Avoid large, heavy meals that may lead to discomfort or

	levels and prevent nausea.	indigestion.
Food Safety	Practice good food safety habits by washing hands, cooking foods thoroughly, and storing food properly.	Avoid consuming undercooked or raw foods, especially when the immune system is compromised.
Individualized Approach	Work with a registered dietitian or healthcare professional to tailor nutrition strategies to your specific needs.	Avoid making dietary changes without proper guidance or medical advice.

For cancer patients, it is important to avoid processed and sugary foods, because processed and sugary foods can cause inflammation and increase the risk of weight gain, which can negatively impact a cancer patient's health and recovery. In the meantime, cancer patients may experience changes in their sense of taste and smell, which can make food less appealing. Therefore, using herbs and spices to add flavor to food can make it more appetizing and enjoyable to eat.

Nutrition Strategies for Cancer Treatment Side Effects

Cancer treatments such as chemotherapy, radiation therapy, and surgery can cause a range of side effects that can impact a patient's ability to eat and maintain proper nutrition. Here are some nutrition strategies that may be helpful for cancer patients who are experiencing treatment side effects:

1. Nausea and Vomiting: Nausea and vomiting are common side effects of cancer treatment and can make it difficult to eat and

maintain proper nutrition. To help alleviate these symptoms, it may be helpful to eat small, frequent meals throughout the day rather than three large meals. Patients should avoid eating their favorite foods during periods of nausea and vomiting, as they may develop an aversion to these foods in the future. Foods that are high in protein, such as lean meats, poultry, fish, and eggs, may be easier to tolerate and can help promote healing. Foods that are easy to digest, such as crackers, toast, and white rice, can help settle the stomach. Ginger, which can be consumed as tea or in capsule form, has been shown to have anti-nausea properties.

2. Taste Changes: Cancer treatments can also cause changes in taste, which can make it difficult to enjoy certain foods. Patients may find that they have a metallic or bitter taste in their mouth, or that their sense of taste is dull. To help alleviate these symptoms, it may be helpful to experiment with different flavors and seasonings to make food more appealing. Patients may also find that cold or room-temperature foods are easier to tolerate than hot foods.

3. Mouth Sores: Chemotherapy and radiation therapy can cause mouth sores, which can make it painful to eat and drink. Patients should avoid acidic or spicy foods, as these can irritate the sores. Soft, bland foods such as mashed potatoes, yogurt, and scrambled eggs may be easier to tolerate. Patients should also avoid alcohol and tobacco, which can further irritate the sores.

4. Diarrhea: Diarrhea is another common side effect of cancer treatment and can lead to dehydration and malnutrition. Patients should avoid high-fiber foods (raw fruits and vegetables, whole grains), greasy or fried foods, and foods that are very sweet or very salty. Instead, they should focus on low-fiber, easily digestible foods such as white rice, bananas, apple sauce and boiled potatoes. Drinking plenty of fluids, such as water, sports drinks, and clear broths, can help prevent dehydration. Probiotics, which are beneficial bacteria found in yogurt and other fermented foods, may also help alleviate

diarrhea.

5. Fatigue: Cancer treatment can cause fatigue, which can make it difficult to prepare meals and eat regularly. Patients should focus on nutrient-dense foods that require minimal preparation, such as canned soups, frozen meals, and pre-cut fruits and vegetables. Patients may also find it helpful to enlist the help of friends and family members to prepare meals and provide support.

6. Constipation: Cancer patients may also experience constipation as a side effect of treatment. To alleviate constipation, cancer patients should consume foods that are high in fiber, such as whole grains, fruits, and vegetables. Drinking plenty of fluids can also help prevent constipation.

If a cancer patient is experiencing any of the side effects, the patient should work with a registered dietitian to make nutritional plans with the side effects in consideration. By focusing on nutrient-dense, easily digestible foods and avoiding foods that exacerbate treatment side effects, cancer patients can help ensure that they are receiving the nutrition they need to support their overall health and well-being.

Liquid Nutritional Foods for Cancer Patients

Certain side effects from cancer treatments can make it difficult for a cancer patient to eat solid foods. These side effects may include mouth sores, difficulty swallowing, nausea, vomiting, or a loss of appetite. Liquid nutritional foods can provide a high amount of calories, protein, and other essential nutrients in a small volume, making it easier for patients to consume enough nutrition. It is important to note that liquid nutritional foods should not replace whole foods entirely; whenever possible, a balanced diet with a variety of fresh, whole foods is encouraged. On the other hand, liquid nutritional foods can be a valuable addition to the diet of cancer patients, and there are a variety of liquid nutrition options available, including meal replacement drinks, protein shakes, and soups. By considering nutrient content, caloric intake, flavor and texture, digestibility, and medical considerations, healthcare providers and caregivers can help ensure that the patient is receiving adequate nutrition to support their overall health and well-being.

The table below summarizes why a cancer patient should consider liquid nutritional foods and provides dos and don'ts for their consumption.

Reason to Consider Liquid Nutritional Foods	Dos	Don'ts
Ease of Consumption	Opt for meal replacement shakes, smoothies, or liquid supplements that are easy to consume.	Don't rely solely on liquid foods if you are able to tolerate solid foods without discomfort.
Nutritional Support	Choose liquid nutritional foods that are nutrient-dense and provide a balance of proteins, carbohydrates, healthy fats, vitamins, and minerals.	Avoid liquid foods that are high in added sugars or lack essential nutrients.
Weight Maintenance or Gain	Select calorie-dense liquid nutritional foods to support weight maintenance or gain.	Don't rely solely on liquid foods if you need to lose weight or if they do not align with your nutritional goals.
Hydration Support	Include liquid nutritional foods that provide hydration along with essential nutrients.	Don't rely solely on liquid foods for hydration if you can consume adequate fluids from other sources.
Digestive Support	Opt for easily digestible liquid nutritional foods	Avoid liquid foods that exacerbate

	that are gentle on the digestive system.	digestive issues or discomfort.
Convenience and Portability	Choose ready-to-drink liquid nutritional options or powders that can be easily mixed with water or other liquids.	Don't solely rely on liquid foods if you can tolerate and access a variety of whole foods.

Liquid nutritional foods can be a helpful way to increase caloric intake for cancer patients who are struggling to eat enough to maintain their weight. Be sure to choose products that provide enough calories to meet the patient's needs, based on their age, gender, weight, and activity level. Some liquid nutrition products may be easier to digest than others. Consider choosing options that are low in fat and fiber, which can be harder for the body to digest. It may also be helpful to choose products that are lactose-free or gluten-free if the patient has any intolerances or sensitivities. In addition to commercial liquid nutrition products, there are also homemade options that can be tailored to the patient's preferences and nutritional needs. For example, smoothies made with fruits, vegetables, and protein powders can be a great way to incorporate a variety of nutrients into the patient's diet. Soups and broths made with nutrient-rich ingredients such as bone broth, vegetables, and lean proteins can also be a good option.

Before incorporating liquid nutrition into a cancer patient's diet, it is important to consult with their healthcare provider to ensure that it is safe and appropriate. Some cancer treatments or medications may interact with certain liquid nutrition products, or the patient may have other medical conditions that need to be taken into consideration.

Here is a table listing some popular commercial brands of liquid nutrition foods along with brief descriptions.

Brand	Description	Website
Ensure	Ensure offers a range of liquid nutritional drinks that provide balanced nutrition and various flavors (vanilla, chocolate, strawberry etc). They cater to different dietary needs and offer options for specific health conditions.	ensure.com
Boost	Boost provides a selection of ready-to-drink liquid nutritional beverages with different formulations and flavors. They focus on providing essential nutrients and extra calories for weight gain.	boost.com
Orgain	Orgain offers a variety of organic, plant-based liquid nutrition products, including ready-to-drink shakes and powders. Their products are formulated with high-quality ingredients and are available in different flavors.	orgain.com
Soylent	Soylent provides meal replacement shakes and drinks designed to provide balanced nutrition. Their products are plant-based and come in different formulations, including options for specific dietary needs.	soylent.com
Nutricia Fortisip	Nutricia Fortisip offers a range of liquid nutritional supplements designed for people with increased nutritional needs. They provide a comprehensive mix of	nutricia.co.uk

	essential nutrients and are available in various flavors.	
Kate Farms	Kate Farms offers plant-based, organic, and allergen-friendly liquid meal replacement shakes and formulas. Their products are designed to provide complete nutrition and are available in different formulations.	katefarms.com
Glucerna	Glucerna specializes in liquid nutritional products for people with diabetes. They provide shakes and beverages formulated to help manage blood sugar levels while providing balanced nutrition.	glucerna.com
ProNourish	ProNourish offers low FODMAP, gluten-free, and lactose-free nutritional drinks formulated for individuals with digestive sensitivities. They provide a blend of essential nutrients and are available in different flavors.	pronourish.com
Carnation Breakfast Essentials	Carnation Breakfast Essentials offers ready-to-drink nutritional beverages that are often consumed as breakfast replacements. They contain essential nutrients and are available in various flavors.	carnationbreakfastessentials.com

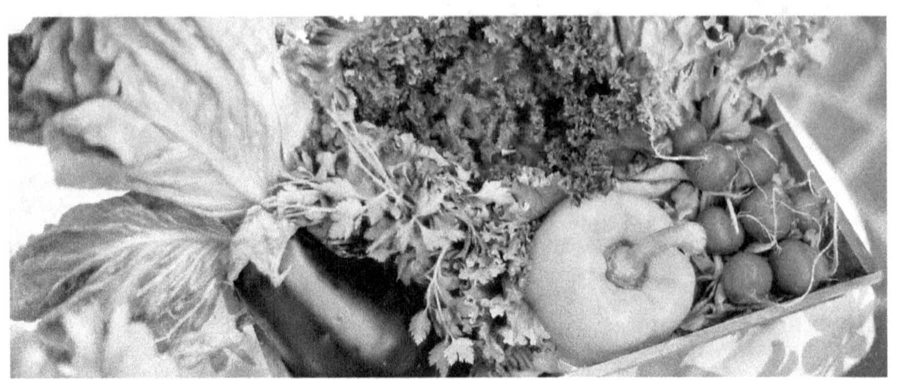

CHAPTER 12 ANTI-INFLAMMATORY DIET, DASH DIET, MEDITERRANEAN DIET AND VEGETARIAN DIET

An anti-inflammatory diet is a dietary approach aimed at reducing chronic inflammation in the body. Chronic inflammation is a contributing factor to many medical conditions, such as heart disease, diabetes, arthritis, and cancer. The anti-inflammatory diet focuses on consuming whole, nutrient-dense foods that can help reduce inflammation and promote overall health. For example, cancer patients can focus on consuming foods that are high in antioxidants such as berries and leafy greens while limiting intake of processed and red meat. Also, a cancer patient may have other medical conditions which can benefit from an anti-inflammatory diet as well. The below table lists the major reasons why a cancer patient should consider an anti-inflammatory diet as part of a comprehensive treatment plan.

Reasons to Consider an Anti-Inflammatory Diet	Description

Reduce Chronic Inflammation	An anti-inflammatory diet focuses on consuming foods that help lower inflammation in the body, which may be beneficial for overall health and potentially impact the cancer microenvironment.
Support Immune Function	The diet includes nutrient-rich foods that support immune function, providing the body with vitamins, minerals, and antioxidants that can help fight infections and potentially enhance defense against cancer cells.
Promote Healthy Weight	An anti-inflammatory diet typically emphasizes whole, unprocessed foods, which can help maintain a healthy weight or support weight loss efforts when needed. This can be important, as excess weight is linked to an increased risk of certain cancers and poorer treatment outcomes.
Reduce Oxidative Stress	The diet is often rich in antioxidants, which help neutralize free radicals and reduce oxidative stress. By consuming antioxidant-rich foods, cancer patients may help minimize DNA damage caused by oxidative stress.

Support Digestive Health	An anti-inflammatory diet includes fiber-rich foods, probiotics, and healthy fats, which can support digestive health and alleviate gastrointestinal side effects that may arise from cancer treatments.
Enhance Overall Well-being	Following an anti-inflammatory diet can contribute to overall well-being, providing more energy, better nutrition, and a sense of control over one's diet and health during cancer treatment.

Principles and Benefits of an Anti-Inflammatory Diet

The table below summarizes the principles and benefits of an anti-inflammatory diet

Principles of an Anti-Inflammatory Diet	Benefits
Emphasize Whole, Unprocessed Foods	Provides a rich array of vitamins, minerals, and antioxidants that support overall health and well-being.
Increase Consumption of Fruits and Vegetables	Provides a wide range of phytochemicals, antioxidants, and fiber that help reduce inflammation and support

	immune function.
Choose Healthy Fats	Includes sources of healthy fats, such as olive oil, nuts, seeds, and fatty fish, which have anti-inflammatory properties and support heart health.
Opt for Lean Proteins	Prioritizes lean protein sources like fish, poultry, legumes, and tofu, which offer essential amino acids and help reduce inflammation.
Minimize Processed and Sugary Foods	Reduces consumption of foods that can contribute to inflammation and may have negative health effects.
Limit Saturated and Trans Fats	Reduces intake of fats that can promote inflammation and have adverse effects on heart health.
Include Anti-Inflammatory Spices and Herbs	Incorporates spices and herbs like turmeric, ginger, garlic, and rosemary, which possess anti-inflammatory properties.
Stay Hydrated	Promotes hydration with water, herbal teas, and other fluids, which aids in the removal of toxins and supports overall health.
Practice Mindful Eating	Encourages mindful eating to develop a healthy relationship with food and improve digestion and absorption of nutrients.

List of foods to include or avoid in an anti-inflammatory diet

Here is a table listing specific foods that should be included and avoided in an anti-inflammatory diet for cancer patients.

Foods to Include in an Anti-Inflammatory Diet	Examples
Fruits and Vegetables	Berries, leafy greens, broccoli, tomatoes, bell peppers, citrus fruits, cherries, sweet potatoes, etc.
Healthy Fats	Olive oil, avocados, nuts (almonds, walnuts), seeds (flaxseeds, chia seeds), fatty fish (salmon, mackerel)
Lean Proteins	Fish, poultry (skinless), legumes (beans, lentils), tofu, tempeh
Whole Grains	Quinoa, brown rice, whole wheat bread and pasta, oats
Herbs and Spices	Turmeric, ginger, garlic, cinnamon, rosemary, oregano
Nuts and Seeds	Almonds, walnuts, flaxseeds, chia seeds
Green Tea	Provides antioxidants and anti-inflammatory compounds
Probiotic-Rich Foods	Yogurt (unsweetened), kefir, sauerkraut, kimchi

Plenty of Water	Hydration is crucial for overall health and to flush out toxins

Foods to Avoid in an Anti-Inflammatory Diet	Examples
Processed and Packaged Foods	Fast food, frozen meals, chips, sugary cereals, processed meats
Refined Grains	White bread, white rice, refined pasta
Sugary Foods and Beverages	Soda, candy, desserts, sugary drinks, sweetened cereals
Saturated and Trans Fats	Butter, margarine, high-fat meats, full-fat dairy products, fried foods
Excessive Alcohol	Limit alcohol intake or avoid it altogether, as it can promote inflammation and compromise immune function
High Sodium Foods	Processed snacks, canned soups, fast food, salty snacks
Red and Processed Meats	Beef, pork, bacon, hot dogs, sausages
Artificial Additives and Preservatives	Artificial sweeteners, food colorings, flavor enhancers
Deep-Fried Foods	French fries, fried chicken, onion rings
Sugary Condiments and Sauces	Ketchup, barbecue sauce, sweetened salad dressings

Note that while frozen meals with high fat, salt and calorie counts should be avoided, it doesn't mean that all frozen foods are bad. In fact, some frozen foods can be easily integrated into a cancer patient's anti-inflammatory diet, especially the ones that are minimally processed, free from additives and preservatives, and rich in nutrients. Here are some examples of acceptable frozen foods that can be included in an anti-inflammatory diet for cancer patients:

1. Frozen Fruits and Vegetables: Choose options without added sugars or sauces. Examples include frozen berries, spinach, kale, broccoli, cauliflower, and mixed vegetable blends.

2. Frozen Seafood: Opt for wild-caught fish and seafood options, such as salmon, sardines, mackerel, shrimp, or scallops. These provide omega-3 fatty acids, which have anti-inflammatory properties.

3. Frozen Legumes: Look for frozen options like edamame, green peas, or chickpeas. They are excellent sources of plant-based protein, fiber, and other beneficial nutrients.

4. Frozen Whole Grains: Choose frozen whole grain options like quinoa, brown rice, or whole grain bread. These can be a convenient source of fiber and complex carbohydrates.

5. Frozen Herbs: Some brands offer frozen herbs like basil, cilantro, or parsley. These can be handy to add flavor and anti-inflammatory compounds to your meals.

6. Frozen Vegetable Burgers: Check for plant-based frozen burger patties made with whole food ingredients and minimal additives. Look for options with vegetables,

legumes, and whole grains as the main ingredients.

7. Frozen Yogurt or Kefir: Choose unsweetened frozen yogurt or kefir that is low in added sugars. These can be beneficial for gut health and provide probiotics.

DASH diet

The Dietary Approaches to Stop Hypertension (DASH) diet is a dietary approach designed to help lower blood pressure and improve overall cardiovascular health. The DASH diet emphasizes consuming whole, nutrient-dense foods while limiting processed and high-sodium foods. The DASH diet encourages consuming a variety of fruits, vegetables, whole grains, lean proteins, and low-fat dairy products. It also emphasizes limiting sodium, saturated and trans fats, and added sugars. Although the DASH diet is not specifically tailored to cancer treatment or prevention, its emphasis on nutrient-rich, whole foods, and healthy eating patterns aligns with general recommendations for supporting overall health and well-being, which can be beneficial for cancer patients, especially ones who also have high blood pressure.

Here is a table showing how the DASH (Dietary Approaches to Stop Hypertension) diet can benefit cancer patients.

DASH Diet Benefits for Cancer Patients
Provides Nutrient-Rich Foods: The DASH diet emphasizes fruits, vegetables, whole grains, lean proteins, and low-fat dairy products, which are rich in essential nutrients that support overall health and immune function.
Promotes Healthy Weight: The DASH diet encourages portion control and limits high-calorie and processed foods, which can help cancer patients maintain a healthy weight. Excess weight is associated with increased cancer risk and poorer outcomes.

High in Antioxidants: The DASH diet includes a variety of fruits, vegetables, and whole grains, which are abundant in antioxidants. Antioxidants help combat oxidative stress, reduce inflammation, and protect cells from damage.

Rich in Fiber: The DASH diet is high in fiber from whole grains, fruits, and vegetables. Adequate fiber intake supports digestive health, helps maintain bowel regularity, and may reduce the risk of certain cancers, such as colorectal cancer.

Low in Sodium: The DASH diet restricts sodium intake, which is beneficial for cancer patients undergoing treatments that may cause fluid retention or affect blood pressure. Lowering sodium intake can help manage these side effects.

Heart-Healthy: The DASH diet is designed to lower blood pressure and improve cardiovascular health. Cancer patients may have an increased risk of heart-related complications, and following a heart-healthy diet can have a positive impact on overall well-being.

Balanced Macronutrients: The DASH diet promotes a balance of carbohydrates, proteins, and healthy fats, which provide energy and support various bodily functions, including tissue repair and immune system functioning.

Reduces Processed Foods: The DASH diet discourages processed and high-sugar foods, which often lack essential nutrients and may contribute to inflammation. Minimizing these foods can be beneficial for cancer patients seeking an anti-inflammatory diet.

Emphasizes Whole Foods: The DASH diet focuses on whole, unprocessed foods, which tend to be more nutrient-dense and provide a wide range of health-promoting compounds, including vitamins, minerals, and phytochemicals.

Mediterranean Diet

The Mediterranean diet is a dietary pattern inspired by the traditional eating habits of countries bordering the Mediterranean Sea, such as Greece, Italy, and Spain. It is characterized by a high consumption of fruits, vegetables, legumes, whole grains, nuts, seeds, olive oil, and herbs and spices. It also includes moderate consumption of fish, seafood, poultry, eggs, and dairy products, while red meat and processed foods are limited.

Dos of the Mediterranean Diet:

1. Eat plenty of fruits and vegetables: Aim for a variety of colorful fruits and vegetables, as they are rich in vitamins, minerals, and antioxidants.

2. Include whole grains: Opt for whole grain bread, pasta, rice, and cereals, which provide fiber and important nutrients.

3. Consume healthy fats: Use extra virgin olive oil as the primary source of fat, and incorporate sources of healthy fats like nuts, seeds, and fatty fish.

4. Prioritize plant-based proteins: Include legumes (beans, lentils, chickpeas) and nuts as sources of protein, and limit red meat consumption.

5. Eat fish and seafood: Include fatty fish like salmon, mackerel, and sardines, which are rich in omega-3 fatty acids.

6. Use herbs and spices: Enhance the flavor of your meals with herbs and spices instead of relying on salt.

7. Stay hydrated: Drink plenty of water throughout the day to maintain hydration.

Don'ts of the Mediterranean Diet:

1. Limit red meat: Red meat should be consumed in moderation. Instead, focus on plant-based protein sources.

2. Reduce processed foods: Minimize consumption of processed foods, such as sugary snacks, sodas, and packaged meals.

3. Limit added sugars: Avoid or limit foods and beverages that contain added sugars, such as sweets, sugary drinks, and desserts.

4. Reduce refined grains: Choose whole grains over refined grains, such as white bread, white rice, and refined cereals.

Now, here is a table illustrating how the Mediterranean diet can benefit cancer patients.

Mediterranean Diet Benefits for Cancer Patients
Abundance of Antioxidants: The Mediterranean diet is rich in fruits, vegetables, and olive oil, providing a wide array of antioxidants that help protect cells from damage caused by free radicals.
Anti-Inflammatory Effects: The diet's emphasis on whole foods, healthy fats (like omega-3s from fish), and phytochemical-rich ingredients can help reduce inflammation, which is linked to the development and progression of cancer.
High Fiber Content: The diet includes ample fiber from fruits, vegetables, legumes, and whole grains, which supports digestion, aids in weight management, and may lower the risk of certain cancers, such as colorectal cancer.

Healthy Fats and Omega-3s: Consuming monounsaturated fats from olive oil, nuts, and seeds, along with omega-3 fatty acids from fatty fish, may help reduce the risk of cancer and promote heart health.

Nutrient-Dense Foods: The Mediterranean diet provides essential vitamins, minerals, and other nutrients from a variety of whole foods, supporting overall health and bolstering the immune system.

Balanced Eating Pattern: The diet encourages a balanced approach to eating, incorporating a wide range of food groups in moderation, which can support energy levels and maintain a healthy weight.

Heart-Healthy Benefits: The Mediterranean diet's emphasis on olive oil, whole grains, and lean protein sources can contribute to cardiovascular health, important for cancer patients undergoing treatments that may affect the heart.

Cultural and Social Aspects: The Mediterranean diet promotes mindful eating and enjoying meals with family and friends, fostering a positive relationship with food and potentially reducing stress levels.

Vegetarian Diet

A vegetarian diet is a dietary pattern that excludes meat, poultry, and seafood. However, there are different types of vegetarian diets, including lacto-vegetarian (includes dairy products), ovo-vegetarian (includes eggs), lacto-ovo vegetarian (includes both dairy products and eggs), and vegan (excludes all animal products). Vegetarian diets typically emphasize plant-based foods such as fruits, vegetables, whole grains, legumes, nuts, and seeds. Following a vegetarian diet can be a healthy dietary approach for cancer patients. However, it is important to ensure that the vegetarian diet is nutritionally balanced and provides the necessary nutrients required during cancer treatment.

Dos of a Vegetarian Diet:

1. Include a variety of plant-based foods: Consume a wide range of fruits, vegetables, whole grains, legumes, nuts, and seeds to obtain a diverse array of nutrients.

2. Focus on plant-based protein sources: Incorporate protein-rich foods such as legumes (beans, lentils, chickpeas), tofu, tempeh, seitan, and edamame.

3. Choose whole grains: Opt for whole grains like quinoa, brown rice, whole wheat bread, and oats, which provide fiber, vitamins, and minerals.

4. Include sources of healthy fats: Consume plant-based fats from sources such as avocados, nuts, seeds, and olive oil.

5. Pay attention to nutrient intake: Ensure adequate intake of essential nutrients like vitamin B12, iron, zinc, calcium, and omega-3 fatty acids through fortified foods or supplements if needed.

6. Consider supplementing with vitamin B12: Vitamin B12 is primarily found in animal products and may be lacking in a vegetarian diet. Cancer patients may require additional vitamin B12 to support their immune system and help with fatigue. Consider supplementing with vitamin B12 or consuming fortified foods such as plant-based milks and breakfast cereals.

7. Stay hydrated: Drink sufficient water throughout the day to maintain hydration.

Don'ts of a Vegetarian Diet:

1. Avoid meat, poultry, and seafood: Exclude these animal-based products from your diet.

2. Limit processed foods: Minimize consumption of processed vegetarian foods, which can be high in added sugars, unhealthy fats, and sodium.

3. Watch out for nutrient deficiencies: Pay attention to nutrients that may be lacking in a vegetarian diet, such as vitamin B12, iron, zinc, calcium, and omega-3 fatty acids. Consider appropriate supplementation or fortified foods if necessary.

4. Avoid excessive reliance on refined carbohydrates: Choose whole grains over refined grains to maintain stable blood sugar levels and ensure adequate fiber intake.

And here is a table illustrating how a vegetarian diet can benefit cancer patients.

Vegetarian Diet Benefits for Cancer Patients
High in Antioxidants: A vegetarian diet rich in fruits, vegetables, and plant-based foods provides a wide array of antioxidants, which help protect cells from damage and reduce the risk of cancer development.
Abundance of Fiber: Plant-based foods in a vegetarian diet are typically high in fiber, which supports healthy digestion, helps maintain bowel regularity, and may lower the risk of certain cancers, such as colorectal cancer.
Healthy Weight Management: Vegetarian diets tend to be lower in calories and saturated fats, making them helpful for maintaining a healthy weight, which is crucial for cancer prevention and management.
Reduced Inflammation: Plant-based diets have shown

anti-inflammatory effects, which can help reduce chronic inflammation associated with cancer development and progression.

Nutrient-Dense Foods: A well-planned vegetarian diet can provide ample amounts of essential vitamins, minerals, and phytochemicals from a variety of plant-based sources, supporting overall health and immune function.

Heart Health Benefits: Vegetarian diets, particularly those low in saturated fats and cholesterol, can promote cardiovascular health, which is important for cancer patients undergoing treatments that may affect the heart.

Potential Reduction in Cancer Risk: Some research suggests that vegetarian diets may be associated with a lower risk of certain types of cancer, including colorectal, breast, and prostate cancer.

Environmental Sustainability: Plant-based diets have a lower carbon footprint and can contribute to environmental sustainability, which may be a consideration for individuals concerned about the environmental impact of food choices.

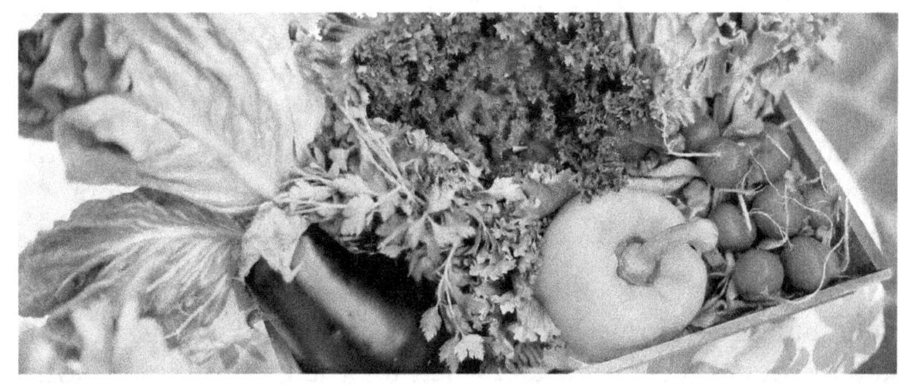

CHAPTER 13 NUTRITION THAT CAN BOOST ONE'S IMMUNE SYSTEM

Having or building a strong immune system is critical for a cancer patient due to several reasons. First and foremost, a robust immune system plays a crucial role in recognizing and eliminating cancer cells. Cancer develops when abnormal cells evade the immune system's surveillance and start multiplying uncontrollably. A strong immune system can identify these cancerous cells and mount an effective immune response to eliminate or control their growth.

Additionally, a healthy immune system is vital for cancer patients undergoing treatments such as chemotherapy or radiation therapy, which can weaken the immune system temporarily. These treatments target not only cancer cells but also affect some healthy cells and immune cells. By maintaining a strong immune system, cancer patients are better equipped to withstand the side effects of treatment, recover more quickly, and reduce the risk of infections and complications.

Furthermore, a strong immune system is essential for long-term cancer management and prevention of cancer recurrence. After treatment, cancer survivors need a healthy immune system to prevent the growth and spread of any remaining cancer cells.

By adopting a healthy lifestyle, including proper nutrition, regular exercise with moderate-intensity activities (walking, swimming, cycling), adequate sleep, and stress management (mindfulness meditation, deep breathing exercises, relaxation), cancer patients can support their immune system and improve their overall well-being.

In this chapter, we will focus on nutritional foods that can help build a strong immune system, for example, several key nutrients have been identified for their immune-boosting properties. Vitamin C is a powerful antioxidant found in citrus fruits, strawberries, and leafy greens, which helps enhance immune cell function. Vitamin D, commonly obtained through sunlight exposure and fatty fish, supports immune regulation. Zinc, abundant in lean meats, legumes, and seeds, assists in immune cell development and function. Probiotics, present in yogurt and fermented foods, promote a healthy gut microbiome, thereby enhancing immune responses. Antioxidant-rich foods, such as berries, nuts, and vegetables, provide a range of vitamins and minerals that support immune function. A well-rounded diet with a variety of nutrient-dense foods rich in fruits, vegetables, whole grains, lean proteins, and healthy fats can contribute to a robust immune system.

Preparing one's own meals from grocery shopping to boost one's immune system

Preparing one's own meals from grocery shopping offers several advantages over relying on restaurant meals or fast foods when it comes to building a cancer patient's immune system. Firstly, cooking at home provides greater control over the ingredients used, allowing for healthier choices. Cancer patients can prioritize nutrient-dense foods such as fresh fruits, vegetables, whole grains, and lean proteins, which are essential for supporting immune function. They can also minimize the intake of unhealthy additives like excessive salt, unhealthy fats, and artificial preservatives commonly found in restaurant or fast-food meals.

Additionally, home-cooked meals enable customization to cater to specific dietary needs or restrictions. Cancer patients may have unique nutritional requirements based on their treatment plans or specific health conditions. By preparing meals at home, they can tailor recipes to incorporate specific immune-boosting foods or avoid ingredients that may negatively impact their health.

Moreover, cooking at home promotes mindful eating and portion control. It allows individuals to pay closer attention to their food choices, portion sizes, and cooking methods. This can be particularly beneficial for cancer patients who may need to maintain a healthy weight and manage potential side effects of treatment, such as nausea or digestive issues.

Overall, preparing one's own meals from grocery shopping empowers cancer patients to make informed dietary choices, prioritize nutrient-rich ingredients, and adapt recipes to their specific needs. It enhances the quality of their diet, supports immune health, and contributes to their overall well-being during cancer treatment and recovery.

Here's a table listing examples of nutrient-dense foods that are critical for a cancer patient's immune system.

Food Group	Examples
Fruits	Berries (blueberries, strawberries), citrus fruits (oranges, grapefruits), kiwi, apples, pomegranate, avocado
Vegetables	Leafy greens (spinach, kale), broccoli, carrots, bell peppers, tomatoes, sweet potatoes, cruciferous vegetables (cauliflower, Brussels sprouts)

Whole Grains	Quinoa, brown rice, oats, whole wheat bread, whole grain pasta, barley
Lean Proteins	Skinless chicken or turkey breast, fish (salmon, tuna), beans, lentils, tofu, Greek yogurt
Nuts and Seeds	Almonds, walnuts, flaxseeds, chia seeds, pumpkin seeds
Healthy Fats	Olive oil, avocado, nuts (almonds, walnuts), seeds (flaxseeds, chia seeds), fatty fish (salmon, mackerel)
Dairy or Alternatives	Low-fat milk, Greek yogurt, cottage cheese, almond milk
Herbs and Spices	Turmeric, ginger, garlic, oregano, cinnamon, rosemary

Ready-to-eat dishes, snacks and liquid foods to boost one's immune system

Ready-to-eat dishes, snacks, and liquid foods can offer several advantages for cancer patients looking to boost their immune system. Firstly, they provide convenience and ease, particularly for individuals who may experience fatigue or have limited energy for meal preparation. Ready-to-eat options save time and effort, allowing cancer patients to focus on their recovery and overall well-being.

Additionally, these foods can be specifically formulated to be nutrient-dense and designed to support immune health. They are often carefully crafted to provide a balance of essential vitamins, minerals, antioxidants, and other beneficial nutrients. Moreover, they can be tailored to address specific dietary needs or restrictions, such as low sodium, high fiber, or lactose-free options. This can be particularly useful for individuals with compromised appetites or digestive issues.

However, it's important to note that not all ready-to-eat options are equally nutritious. Reading labels and choosing products that are minimally processed, low in added sugars, and rich in whole food ingredients is key. Ready-to-eat foods should be considered as a supplement to a balanced diet, and it's still beneficial to incorporate fresh, whole foods whenever possible.

Here are some examples of ready-to-eat dishes, snacks, and liquid foods that can help boost the immune system:

1. Soups: Soups are a great way to incorporate nutrient-dense foods such as vegetables, beans, and lean proteins into your diet. Soups can be made in advance and stored in the refrigerator or freezer for easy reheating. Chicken noodle soup is a classic example of a soup that is rich in immune-boosting nutrients.

2. Smoothies: Smoothies are a convenient way to pack in a variety of immune-boosting nutrients such as fruits, vegetables, and yogurt. Adding spinach, kale, or other leafy greens to a smoothie can provide essential vitamins and antioxidants.

3. Yogurt: Yogurt is a great source of probiotics, which are beneficial bacteria that can help improve gut health and boost the immune system. Greek yogurt is a particularly good choice as it is high in protein and low in sugar.

4. Trail mix: Trail mix is a convenient snack that is rich in immune-boosting nutrients such as nuts and seeds. Almonds, walnuts, and pumpkin seeds are all good choices for a trail mix that is rich in antioxidants and essential nutrients.

5. Hummus: Hummus is a tasty dip that is made from chickpeas, tahini, and olive oil. Chickpeas are a good source of protein and fiber, while olive oil provides healthy fats and antioxidants. Hummus can be paired with vegetables, crackers, or pita bread for a healthy snack.

6. Green tea: Green tea is a rich source of antioxidants and other beneficial compounds that can help boost the immune system. Drinking green tea on a regular basis can help improve overall health and reduce the risk of chronic diseases.

7. Bone broth: Bone broth is a rich source of nutrients such as collagen, gelatin, and amino acids. These nutrients can help support gut health and boost the immune system. Bone broth can be consumed as a hot beverage or used as a base for soups and stews.

Frozen meals and breakfast options to incorporate immune-boosting nutrients

Frozen foods can also be a convenient addition for a cancer patient to add immune-boosting nutrients in breakfasts and meals. For example, frozen vegetable stir-fry can have a variety of immune-boosting nutrients such as Vitamins A and C; frozen wild-caught salmon fillet is rich in omega-3 fatty acids which is anti-inflammatory; frozen blueberries, raspberries and strawberries are a rich source of antioxidants; frozen spinach has iron and other essential nutrients besides Vitamins A and C; frozen whole-grain waffles can be a tasty breakfast option that is rich in fiber and other essential nutrients etc.

Here's a table listing examples of frozen meals and breakfast options with immune-boosting nutrients along with their detailed descriptions.

Type of Food	Examples	Detailed Description
Frozen Meals	Vegetable Stir-Fry with Brown Rice	A frozen meal containing a colorful mix of stir-fried vegetables like broccoli, bell peppers, carrots, and snap peas, served over brown rice. Rich in immune-boosting antioxidants,

		fiber, and vitamins.
	Lemon Herb Baked Salmon with Quinoa	A frozen meal featuring a portion of baked salmon seasoned with lemon and herbs, served alongside a side of quinoa. Provides lean protein, omega-3 fatty acids, and essential minerals like zinc to support immune health.
	Chickpea Curry with Turmeric Rice	A frozen meal consisting of a flavorful chickpea curry made with aromatic spices and served with turmeric-infused rice. Contains plant-based proteins, fiber, and anti-inflammatory properties of turmeric, supporting immune function.
Breakfast Options	Berry and Spinach Smoothie Bowl	A frozen breakfast option comprising a pre-portioned smoothie bowl blend of berries (such as blueberries and strawberries) and spinach. Offers a nutrient-rich combination of antioxidants, vitamins, and fiber for immune support.
	Whole Grain Oatmeal Cups with Nuts and Seeds	Individual servings of frozen oatmeal cups made with whole grains and mixed with a variety of nuts and seeds like almonds, walnuts, flaxseeds, and chia seeds. Provides fiber, healthy fats, and essential nutrients to

| | | fuel the immune system. |
| Veggie Egg White Omelet | | A frozen egg white omelet packed with a medley of colorful vegetables such as bell peppers, onions, and spinach. Offers low-fat protein, vitamins, and minerals necessary for immune function and overall health. |

Restaurant and fast-food options that provide immune-boosting nutrients

While restaurant and fast-food options may not always be the first choice for immune-boosting nutrition, there can still be some advantages for cancer patients seeking to support their immune system. One advantage is the increasing availability of healthier menu choices at many restaurants and fast-food chains. Some establishments offer options that include salads with lean proteins, grilled or roasted vegetables, whole grain wraps or sandwiches, and even plant-based alternatives. These choices can provide essential nutrients, such as vitamins, minerals, fiber, and antioxidants, which are beneficial for immune function.

Another advantage is the convenience and social aspect that restaurants and fast-food options offer. Eating out can provide an opportunity for cancer patients to socialize with friends and family or enjoy a break from cooking and meal preparation. By making informed choices and selecting healthier options, cancer patients can still find dishes that contribute to their overall nutrition and well-being. It's important to prioritize fresh ingredients, lean proteins, whole grains, and vegetables, and to be mindful of portion sizes and added sugars or unhealthy fats commonly found in some restaurants or fast-food meals.

However, it's crucial to note that not all restaurant or fast-food options are equally nutritious, and some can be high in calories, unhealthy fats, sodium, and added sugars. It's advisable to research menu options in advance, choose establishments with healthier offerings, and customize dishes to suit specific dietary needs. Balancing restaurant or fast-food choices with predominantly home-cooked, nutrient-dense meals is recommended for optimal immune support during cancer treatment and recovery.

Some popular restaurant foods with immune-boosting nutrients are grilled chicken or fish, vegetable-packed salads, broth-based soup, sushi rolls made with salmon or tuna, bean burrito or bowl, and Greek yogurt parfait etc. Below is a table with some healthier options available at popular restaurants and fast-food chains that can contribute to a cancer patient's immune system, along with their brief descriptions.

Restaurant	Option	Description
Subway	Veggie Delite Salad	A salad loaded with a variety of fresh vegetables, such as lettuce, tomatoes, cucumbers, peppers, and onions. Can be customized with lean protein options like turkey breast or chicken.
Panera Bread	Mediterranean Veggie Sandwich	A sandwich made with a medley of roasted vegetables, feta cheese, hummus, and fresh greens on whole grain bread. Provides a mix of immune-boosting veggies, fiber, and plant-based proteins.

Chipotle Mexican Grill	Chicken or Sofritas Bowl	A customizable bowl with choices of grilled chicken or sofritas (spicy tofu), combined with brown rice, black beans, fajita veggies, and a variety of toppings like salsa, guacamole, and lettuce. Offers protein, fiber, and vitamins from vegetables.
Sweetgreen	Kale Caesar Salad with Grilled Chicken	A nutrient-packed salad featuring kale, romaine lettuce, grilled chicken, parmesan, and a Caesar dressing made with yogurt or healthier alternatives. Provides a mix of greens, lean protein, and calcium.
Freshii	Teriyaki Twist Bowl	A bowl with a base of brown rice or quinoa, topped with teriyaki-glazed chicken or tofu, and a colorful assortment of vegetables like broccoli, carrots, and edamame. Offers a balance of protein, fiber, and antioxidants.
Blaze Pizza	Build-Your-Own Pizza with Whole Wheat Crust	Customizable pizza with the option to choose a whole wheat crust and load it with various vegetable toppings like mushrooms, peppers, onions, and spinach. Incorporates whole grains and

		immune-boosting veggies.
Noodles & Company	Zucchini Shrimp Scampi	A dish made with zucchini noodles, succulent shrimp, garlic, and a lemony sauce. Provides a low-carb alternative to traditional pasta while offering lean protein and essential nutrients.
P.F. Chang's	Buddha's Feast Stir-Fried Vegetables	A stir-fried medley of vibrant vegetables like bok choy, mushrooms, snow peas, and carrots in a savory sauce. A plant-based option packed with antioxidants, fiber, and vitamins.
Freshii	Superfood Salad	A salad composed of nutrient-rich ingredients like kale, spinach, quinoa, blueberries, almonds, and a lemon vinaigrette. Offers a variety of immune-boosting antioxidants, vitamins, and minerals.
Chipotle Mexican Grill	Salad Bowl with Barbacoa	A salad bowl with barbacoa (slow-cooked shredded beef), mixed greens, black beans, fajita veggies, and a choice of toppings like salsa and guacamole. Provides protein, fiber, and a range of nutrients from vegetables.

Jason's Deli	Turkey Wrap	A wrap made with lean turkey, whole grain tortilla, lettuce, tomatoes, and other fresh vegetables. Offers a balanced combination of protein, whole grains, and immune-boosting veggies.
The Cheesecake Factory	SkinnyLicious Grilled Salmon	Grilled salmon fillet served with fresh vegetables and a side salad. Provides a good source of omega-3 fatty acids, lean protein, and a variety of nutrients from vegetables.
Shake Shack	Veggie Shack	A vegetarian burger made with a patty consisting of black beans, brown rice, and roasted beets, topped with lettuce, tomato, onions, and vegan mayo. Offers plant-based protein and a range of immune-boosting veggies.
Fresh To Order	Turkey Avocado Cobb Salad	A cobb salad featuring turkey breast, avocado, mixed greens, tomatoes, cucumbers, hard-boiled eggs, and a light dressing. Provides a balance of lean protein, healthy fats, and immune-boosting vegetables.
MOD Pizza	MOD Salad	A customizable salad with a choice of greens, toppings like grilled chicken, chickpeas, sun-dried tomatoes, and a

		range of dressings. Offers a mix of protein, fiber, and nutrients from vegetables.

Foods to avoid or limit to support a healthy immune system

Certain foods can have a negative impact on the immune system, particularly for cancer patients who are already dealing with compromised immunity. These foods typically fall into the category of processed or ultra-processed foods (chips, cookies, fried foods etc), which are often high in added sugars, unhealthy fats, and refined carbohydrates. Consuming excessive amounts of these foods can lead to inflammation, weight gain, and the disruption of the body's natural defense mechanisms.

It is crucial for cancer patients to avoid certain foods to support a healthy immune system. High-sugar foods, such as sugary beverages, desserts, and candies, can weaken immune function and promote inflammation. Similarly, foods high in unhealthy fats, such as deep-fried items, processed meats, and high-fat dairy products, can impair immune response and increase the risk of chronic diseases. Additionally, refined carbohydrates like white bread, pasta, and sugary cereals can cause spikes in blood sugar levels and contribute to inflammation. Cancer patients should also avoid excessive alcohol consumption.

Here's a table with examples of processed or ultra-processed foods, including their brand names and brief descriptions.

Food	Brand Name	Description
Soda	Coca-Cola, Pepsi, Sprite, etc.	Carbonated beverages that are high in added sugars and provide empty calories without any nutritional value.
Potato Chips	Lay's, Pringles,	Thin, crispy slices

	Ruffles, etc.	of potatoes that are typically deep-fried and high in unhealthy fats, sodium, and artificial flavors.
Sugary Cereal	Frosted Flakes, Froot Loops, Cocoa Puffs, etc.	Breakfast cereals that are heavily processed, loaded with added sugars, and lack essential nutrients and fiber.
Processed Meats	Oscar Mayer, Hormel, Hillshire Farm, etc.	Meats that have been processed and preserved through methods like smoking, curing, or adding preservatives, often containing high levels of sodium and unhealthy additives.
Frozen Dinners	Lean Cuisine, Stouffer's, Healthy Choice, etc.	Pre-packaged meals that are typically high in sodium, preservatives, and unhealthy fats, while lacking in fresh ingredients and essential nutrients.
Packaged Snack Cakes	Twinkies, Ho Hos, Ding Dongs, etc.	Individually wrapped cakes that are highly processed, loaded with added sugars, unhealthy fats, and artificial ingredients.
Fast Food	McDonald's Big	Hamburgers from

Burgers	Mac, Burger King Whopper, etc.	fast food chains that are often made with processed meat patties, high in unhealthy fats, sodium, and artificial ingredients.
Margarine	Country Crock, I Can't Believe It's Not Butter, etc.	A butter substitute made from vegetable oils, often containing trans fats, artificial additives, and lacking the nutritional benefits of natural butter.
Instant Noodles	Ramen Noodles, Cup Noodles, Maruchan, etc.	Pre-cooked noodles that come with powdered flavor packets, often high in sodium, unhealthy fats, and lacking in essential nutrients.
Flavored Yogurt	Yoplait, Dannon, Chobani Fruit-on-the-Bottom, etc.	Yogurt products that are loaded with added sugars, artificial flavors, and may lack the probiotic benefits of plain, unsweetened yogurt.

These examples highlight some common processed or ultra-processed foods that are often high in added sugars, unhealthy fats, sodium, and artificial additives. It is important for cancer patients to limit their consumption of these foods and opt for whole, unprocessed options that are rich in nutrients and support a healthy immune system.

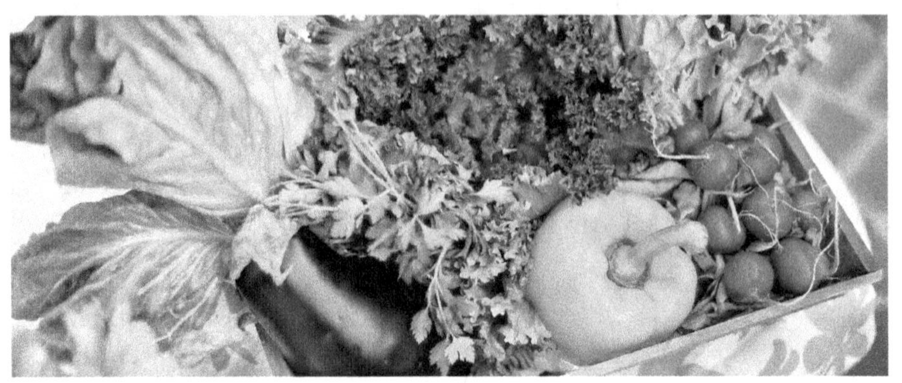

CHAPTER 14 OFF-LABEL DRUG USE FOR CANCER TREATMENT

Off-label drug use refers to the practice of prescribing medications for purposes other than those officially approved by regulatory authorities, such as the Food and Drug Administration (FDA) or European Medicines Agency (EMA). In the context of cancer treatment, off-label drug use may involve using medications that have been approved for other types of cancer or non-cancerous conditions to treat specific types of cancer. This approach can have both pros and cons.

One advantage of off-label drug use in cancer treatment is the potential for expanded treatment options. It allows healthcare providers to explore alternative therapies when standard treatments have failed or are unavailable. It can provide patients with access to potentially beneficial medications that may have shown promise in early studies or anecdotal evidence. Off-label drug use also allows for personalized treatment approaches, tailoring therapy to the unique needs and characteristics of individual patients.

However, there are also drawbacks to off-label drug use. The primary concern is the lack of robust scientific evidence supporting the safety and effectiveness of these medications for specific off-label use. Clinical trials may not have been conducted for the particular cancer type or stage, which can make it difficult to determine the optimal dosage, duration, and potential side effects. Additionally, insurance coverage for off-label drugs can be limited, leading to financial burdens for patients. It is important for healthcare providers to carefully weigh the potential benefits and risks of off-label drug use, thoroughly discuss them with patients, and ensure appropriate informed consent. Rigorous monitoring and close collaboration between the healthcare team and patients are crucial to ensure patient safety and optimize treatment outcomes.

That being said, some off-label drugs have shown promise in the treatment of late-stage cancers. One notable example of off-label use of the drug metformin in cancer treatment is its potential efficacy in patients with breast cancer. While metformin is primarily prescribed to manage type 2 diabetes, studies have suggested that it may have anticancer properties. Several preclinical and observational studies have shown promising results, indicating that metformin may have a beneficial impact on tumor growth and progression.

In the case of breast cancer, laboratory studies have demonstrated that metformin can inhibit cancer cell growth, promote cell death (apoptosis), and suppress the formation of new blood vessels that supply tumors (angiogenesis). Additionally, metformin has been found to affect key signaling pathways involved in cancer development and progression, such as the AMP-activated protein kinase (AMPK) pathway.

Clinical studies investigating the use of metformin in breast cancer have also shown promising outcomes. For instance, a retrospective analysis of breast cancer patients with diabetes found that those taking metformin alongside their cancer treatment had a lower risk of cancer recurrence and improved survival compared to those not taking metformin. Other studies have reported similar findings, suggesting that metformin may enhance the efficacy of standard breast cancer therapies and improve patient outcomes.

One patient success story involves a woman named Caroline, who was diagnosed with stage 4 ovarian cancer. She underwent multiple rounds of chemotherapy and surgery, but her cancer continued to progress. Her oncologist suggested trying metformin off-label as a possible treatment option. Caroline was hesitant at first, but after researching the potential benefits and consulting with her healthcare team, she decided to give it a try. Over the course of several months, Caroline noticed a significant improvement in her symptoms. Her cancer markers began to decrease, and her oncologist reported that her tumors had shrunk. Today, Caroline continues to take metformin in combination with other cancer treatments. While her journey is not over yet, she is grateful for the additional treatment option that metformin has provided and remains hopeful for the future.

It's important to note that while Caroline's story is inspiring, every patient's journey is unique, and the effectiveness of metformin as a cancer treatment may vary depending on the type and stage of cancer. It's essential to work closely with a healthcare professional to determine whether off-label drug use, such as metformin, is appropriate and safe for individual patients.

Below is a table listing some examples of off-label drugs used in the treatment of lung cancer, breast cancer, pancreatic cancer, colon cancer, and prostate cancer, along with their approved use and off-label use.

Drug	Type of Cancer	Approved Use	Off-Label Use
Afatinib	Lung Cancer	EGFR-mutated NSCLC	Other subtypes of lung cancer

Trastuzumab	Breast Cancer	HER2-positive breast cancer	Other settings
FOLFIRINOX	Pancreatic Cancer	N/A	Advanced pancreatic cancer
Regorafenib	Colon Cancer	Colorectal cancer	Other gastrointestinal cancers
Docetaxel	Prostate Cancer	Metastatic prostate cancer	Earlier stages or combination therapies
Osimertinib	Lung Cancer	EGFR-mutated NSCLC	Other EGFR mutations
Everolimus	Breast Cancer	Certain types of breast cancer	Other subtypes
Capecitabine	Pancreatic Cancer	Colorectal cancer	Pancreatic cancer
Cabazitaxel	Prostate Cancer	Metastatic castration-resistant prostate cancer	Other settings
Lapatinib	Breast Cancer	HER2-positive breast cancer	Different combinations or settings
Panitumumab	Colon Cancer	KRAS wild-type colorectal cancer	Other subsets of colon cancer patients
Alectinib	Lung Cancer	ALK-positive NSCLC	ROS1-positive lung cancer
TAS-102	Colon Cancer	Colorectal cancer	Refractory cases
Radium-223	Prostate Cancer	Bone metastases in castration-resistant prostate cancer	Specific cases
Olaparib	Pancreatic Cancer	Ovarian and breast cancer	Pancreatic cancer with specific genetic mutations

And here is a table listing some examples of off-label drugs used in cancer treatment, along with their approved use, detailed description of off-label use, and possible mechanisms.

Drug	Approved Use	Off-Label Use	Possible Mechanism
Metformin	Type 2 diabetes treatment	Breast cancer treatment	Inhibition of cancer cell growth, apoptosis, and angiogenesis through AMPK pathway modulation.
Aspirin	Pain relief, anti-inflammatory	Colorectal cancer prevention	Inhibition of COX-2 enzyme, reduction of inflammation, and suppression of tumor growth.

Drug	Approved Use	Off-Label Use	Mechanism
Thalidomide	Treatment for leprosy and multiple myeloma	Solid tumor treatment, especially ovarian cancer	Anti-angiogenic effects, modulation of immune response, and inhibition of tumor growth.
Propranolol	Hypertension, cardiac arrhythmias	Infantile hemangioma treatment	Blockade of beta-adrenergic receptors, leading to decreased tumor proliferation and angiogenesis.
Tamoxifen	Breast cancer treatment	Endometrial cancer treatment	Selective estrogen receptor modulator, inhibiting estrogen signaling and preventing cancer cell growth.
Celecoxib	Pain relief, anti-inflammatory	Various cancers, including colorectal, prostate, and lung cancer	COX-2 inhibition, suppression of inflammation, and anti-angiogenic effects.
Rituximab	Non-Hodgkin lymphoma treatment	Chronic lymphocytic leukemia treatment	Targeting CD20 antigen on B cells, leading to cell death and suppression of cancer cell growth.
Bortezomib	Multiple myeloma treatment	Mantle cell lymphoma treatment	Proteasome inhibition, causing cell cycle arrest, apoptosis, and inhibition of tumor growth.
Imatinib	Chronic myeloid leukemia treatment	Gastrointestinal stromal tumor treatment	Inhibition of tyrosine kinases, such as BCR-ABL and c-KIT, disrupting signaling pathways critical for cancer cell growth.
Dexamethasone	Anti-inflammatory, immunosuppressant	Multiple myeloma treatment	Induction of apoptosis, inhibition of angiogenesis, and modulation of immune response.

It's important to note that the off-label use of these drugs should be carefully evaluated by healthcare professionals based on individual patient factors, available evidence, and potential risks and benefits. The decision to use off-label drugs in cancer treatment should be made in consultation with the patient and based on the best available evidence and clinical judgment.

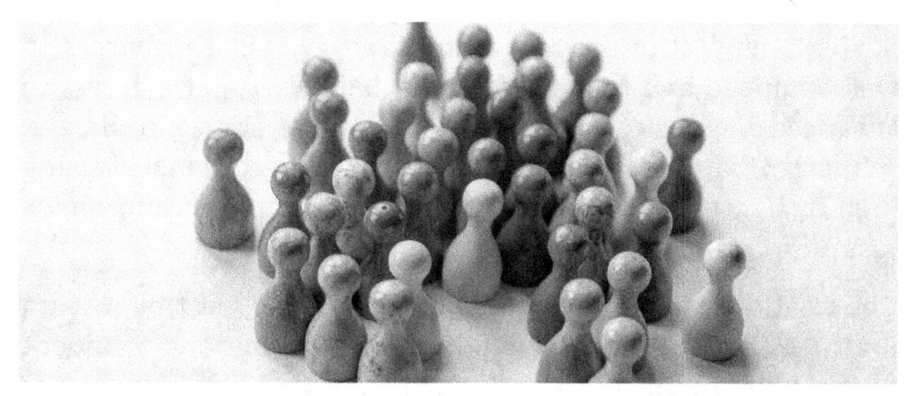

SECTION IV SELECTING THE CANCER TREATMENT TEAM AND TREATMENT CENTER

Choosing a cancer treatment team and facility is a critically important decision for a cancer patient. The quality of care and treatment outcomes can significantly depend on the expertise and experience of the healthcare professionals involved. A cancer treatment team typically consists of various specialists, including oncologists, surgeons, radiologists, and other healthcare professionals, who work together to develop an individualized treatment plan and provide comprehensive care.

First and foremost, the expertise and qualifications of the healthcare professionals are vital. Patients should seek out specialists who have extensive experience and training in their specific type of cancer. The team's collective knowledge and skills can greatly impact treatment decisions, ensuring that the most appropriate and effective therapies are chosen.

Furthermore, the facility where treatment is provided plays a crucial role. Patients should consider factors such as the facility's reputation, accreditation, and available resources. A well-equipped and reputable facility is likely to have access to advanced diagnostic tools, treatment options, clinical trials, and supportive care services. The facility's track record in delivering high-quality care and positive treatment outcomes can provide reassurance and confidence to patients.

The relationship between the patient and the treatment team is also essential. Patients should feel comfortable and confident in their communication with the healthcare professionals, as open and honest dialogue is vital for effective collaboration and shared decision-making. Supportive and compassionate care from the treatment team can greatly contribute to the patient's overall well-being and quality of life throughout the treatment journey.

Ultimately, choosing a knowledgeable and experienced cancer treatment team, as well as a reputable facility, increases the chances of receiving optimal care, personalized treatment plans, and better treatment outcomes for the cancer patient.

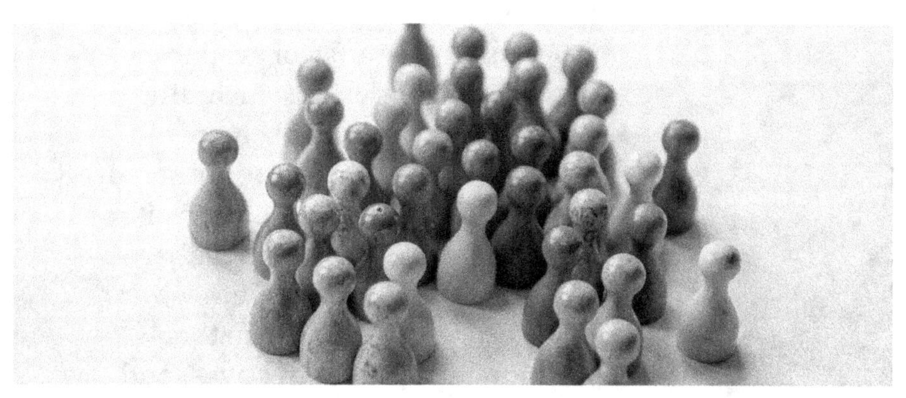

CHAPTER 15 KEY CONSIDERATIONS WHEN SELECTING CANCER TREATMENT TEAM AND FACILITY

The choice of a cancer treatment team and facility should be based on comprehensive research, discussions with healthcare professionals, and personal preferences to ensure the best possible care and treatment outcomes. Below is a table listing key considerations when choosing a cancer treatment team and facility.

Consideration	Details
Expertise	Evaluate the qualifications and experience of the healthcare professionals including oncologists, surgeons, and other specialists on the team, ensuring they specialize in the specific type of cancer. Look for a facility that has experience treating the type of cancer you have.

Treatment Options	Assess the range of available treatment options, including surgery, radiation therapy, chemotherapy, immunotherapy, targeted therapies, etc. Ask if the team offers a personalized treatment plan specific to your needs. Look for a team that communicates effectively and clearly with patients and their families, providing all necessary information about the diagnosis, treatment options, and potential side effects
Research and Trials	Determine if the facility participates in clinical trials or has access to cutting-edge research that may offer additional treatment options.
Support Services	Consider the availability of supportive services like nutritional counseling, emotional support, psychological support, pain management, social work services, palliative care, survivorship programs, and complementary therapies.
Facility Accreditation	Verify if the facility is accredited by reputable organizations that ensure high-quality standards and patient safety, with a good track record for quality care, success rate and patient outcomes.

Reputation and Reviews	Research the facility's reputation and read patient reviews to gain insights into the experiences of others who have received care there.
Location and Travel	Consider the location of the facility in terms of proximity to home, accessibility, and potential travel requirements for treatment visits, including their ability to accommodate your schedule and location. Treatment can be time-consuming and tiring, so choose a location that is convenient and manageable for you.
Insurance Coverage	Check if the facility and treatment team are in-network with your insurance provider to minimize out-of-pocket costs.
Cost and Financial Aid	Evaluate the overall cost of treatment, including potential co-pays, deductibles, and available financial aid or assistance programs.
Communication and Trust	Assess the communication style and level of trust between you and the treatment team, as open and honest dialogue is crucial for effective care.
Personal Preferences	Consider personal preferences such as the size of the facility, availability of private rooms, and the cultural or linguistic needs of the patient.

Ultimately, it's important to choose a cancer treatment team and facility that provides personalized care, takes the time to listen to patient needs and concerns, and offers the most advanced and effective treatment options. Choosing a cancer treatment team and facility is a personal decision that should be made in consultation with your family members/loved ones and healthcare providers. Consider all the factors that are important to you, and don't be afraid to ask questions or seek out additional information to help make an informed decision.

An Oncologist vs a Cancer Treatment Team

When a cancer patient talks about cancer doctors, they tend to think of oncologists, but an oncologist is not the same as a cancer treatment team. An oncologist is a medical specialist who focuses on the diagnosis, treatment, and management of cancer. They are physicians with specialized training in oncology, which is the field of medicine dedicated to the study and treatment of cancer. Oncologists may further specialize in specific areas such as medical oncology (chemotherapy, immunotherapy), radiation oncology (radiation therapy), or surgical oncology (surgical interventions).

On the other hand, a cancer treatment team refers to a multidisciplinary group of healthcare professionals who work together to provide comprehensive care for cancer patients. This team typically includes not only oncologists but also other specialists such as surgeons, radiologists, pathologists, nurses, social workers, and support staff. The cancer treatment team collaborates to develop personalized treatment plans, oversee the patient's care throughout the treatment journey, and address various aspects of the patient's physical, emotional, and psychological well-being.

While an oncologist is an essential member of the cancer treatment team, the team itself encompasses a broader range of professionals who contribute their expertise in different areas of cancer care. The team approach ensures that patients receive comprehensive and coordinated care, with each member bringing their unique perspective and skills to the table. The collaboration and coordination among the team members aim to provide the best possible care and optimize treatment outcomes for cancer patients.

There are several different types of oncologists, each with their own specialized training and responsibilities when treating cancer patients. Here are some of the most common types of oncologists and their responsibilities:

1. Medical Oncologist: A medical oncologist is a doctor who specializes in the diagnosis, treatment, and management of cancer using systemic therapies such as chemotherapy, targeted therapy, and immunotherapy.

2. Radiation Oncologist: A radiation oncologist is a doctor who specializes in the use of radiation therapy to treat cancer. They work closely with other members of the cancer care team to develop and oversee a patient's radiation treatment plan.

3. Surgical Oncologist: A surgical oncologist is a doctor who specializes in the surgical management of cancer. They may perform biopsies, remove tumors, or perform reconstructive surgery following cancer treatment.

4. Pediatric Oncologist: A pediatric oncologist is a doctor who specializes in the diagnosis, treatment, and management of cancer in children. They work closely with other members of the care team to develop and oversee a child's cancer treatment plan.

5. Gynecologic Oncologist: A gynecologic oncologist is a doctor who specializes in the diagnosis and treatment of gynecologic cancers such as ovarian, cervical, and uterine cancer. They may perform surgery, chemotherapy, and other treatments to manage these cancers.

6. Hematologist/Oncologist: A hematologist/oncologist is a doctor who specializes in the diagnosis, treatment, and management of blood cancers such as leukemia, lymphoma, and multiple myeloma. They may use chemotherapy, radiation therapy, or other systemic therapies to treat these cancers.

7. Neuro-Oncologist: A neuro-oncologist is a doctor who specializes in the diagnosis and treatment of cancers of the central nervous system, such as brain tumors. They work closely with other members of the care team to develop and oversee a patient's treatment plan.

Each type of oncologist brings unique skills and expertise to the care team, working together to provide comprehensive, personalized cancer care for patients.

Meanwhile, a cancer treatment team will have many healthcare professionals depending on the type and stage of cancer. Below is a table listing various healthcare professionals commonly found in a cancer treatment team, with each member bringing unique skills and expertise to provide comprehensive, personalized care for cancer patients.

Healthcare Professional	Description
Medical Oncologist	A physician specializing in medical oncology who diagnoses and treats cancer using medications such as chemotherapy, immunotherapy, and targeted therapy. They oversee the overall management of the patient's treatment plan and coordinate care with other members of the team.

Surgical Oncologist	A surgeon specializing in surgical interventions for cancer. They perform procedures such as tumor removal, biopsies, and reconstructive surgeries. Surgical oncologists collaborate with other team members to determine the best surgical approach and ensure comprehensive cancer care.
Radiation Oncologist	A physician specializing in radiation therapy. They use high-energy radiation to target and destroy cancer cells. Radiation oncologists work closely with other team members to develop radiation treatment plans and monitor patients throughout their radiation therapy journey.
Pathologist	A medical doctor who examines tissue samples and cells to diagnose cancer and determine its characteristics. Pathologists play a crucial role in determining the type and stage of cancer, which helps guide treatment decisions. They provide important information for the treatment team to develop personalized care plans.

Radiologist	A physician specializing in medical imaging techniques such as X-rays, CT scans, MRIs, and PET scans. Radiologists interpret imaging results to help diagnose and monitor cancer. They collaborate with other team members to ensure accurate imaging and guide treatment planning and monitoring.
Nurse	Oncology nurses provide direct patient care, administer medications, and monitor patients for side effects and complications. They play a vital role in patient education, support, and coordination of care. Oncology nurses are often the primary point of contact for patients throughout their cancer treatment journey.
Social Worker	Social workers provide emotional support, counseling, and assistance with practical matters such as coordinating community resources, financial aid, and transportation. They help patients and their families navigate the challenges and complexities associated

	with cancer treatment and survivorship.
Palliative Care Specialist	Palliative care specialists focus on improving the quality of life for patients with cancer by managing symptoms, providing pain relief, and addressing physical, emotional, and spiritual needs. They work alongside the treatment team to enhance comfort and support patients and their families during and after treatment.
Genetic Counselor	Genetic counselors assess a patient's risk of inherited cancer predisposition syndromes, provide genetic testing and counseling, and offer recommendations for cancer screening and prevention strategies. They help patients understand their genetic risk factors and make informed decisions regarding their care.
Registered Dietitian	Registered dietitians specialize in nutrition and provide guidance on healthy eating during cancer treatment. They assess nutritional needs, develop

	individualized meal plans, and address side effects that may affect diet. Dietitians help optimize nutrition to support the patient's overall health and well-being.
Psychologist or Psychiatrist	Psychologists or psychiatrists provide mental health support to cancer patients, addressing emotional and psychological aspects of their well-being. They offer counseling, therapy, and support to help patients cope with the challenges and stressors associated with cancer diagnosis, treatment, and survivorship.
Physical Therapist	Physical therapists focus on restoring and improving physical function, mobility, and overall well-being. They help cancer patients manage treatment-related side effects, improve strength and endurance, and enhance quality of life through targeted exercise, manual therapy, and education on self-care techniques.

Let's look at a few examples of cancer treatment teams at several leading cancer centers in the US.

Example: Lung Cancer Treatment Team at Memorial Sloan Kettering Cancer Center (MSKCC)

The lung cancer treatment team at Memorial Sloan Kettering Cancer Center (MSKCC) may include the following healthcare professionals shown in the table below.

Healthcare Professional	Description
Medical Oncologist	Specializes in medical oncology and oversees the medical treatment of lung cancer patients. They develop personalized treatment plans, including chemotherapy, immunotherapy, targeted therapy, or a combination of these, and monitor the patient's response to treatment.
Surgical Oncologist	Expert in performing surgical procedures for lung cancer, such as lobectomy, pneumonectomy, or minimally invasive surgeries like video-assisted thoracoscopic surgery (VATS). They assess the patient's surgical eligibility, perform the procedure, and collaborate with other team members to ensure comprehensive care.
Radiation Oncologist	Specializes in radiation therapy for lung cancer. They

	use advanced techniques such as intensity-modulated radiation therapy (IMRT), stereotactic body radiation therapy (SBRT), or proton therapy to deliver precise radiation to the tumor, while minimizing damage to healthy tissue surrounding the lungs.
Pulmonologist	Focuses on lung health and respiratory diseases. In the context of lung cancer, they play a critical role in diagnosing lung nodules, evaluating lung function, and providing expertise in managing symptoms like shortness of breath or cough. They may perform bronchoscopy or other procedures to gather additional information.
Thoracic Surgeon	A surgical specialist who focuses on diseases affecting the chest, including lung cancer. They collaborate with other team members to determine the appropriate surgical approach, perform complex lung resections, and work towards achieving optimal outcomes for patients undergoing lung

	cancer surgery.
Radiologist	A physician specialized in interpreting medical imaging tests like chest CT scans, PET scans, or MRI scans. They provide detailed reports on the location, size, and characteristics of lung tumors, helping guide treatment decisions and monitor treatment response.
Nurse Navigator	A specialized nurse who serves as a central point of contact, guiding and supporting lung cancer patients throughout their journey. They provide education, coordinate appointments, facilitate communication between healthcare providers, and assist patients in accessing resources and support services.
Oncology Nurse	Registered nurses with expertise in oncology who provide direct patient care, administer medications, monitor treatment side effects, and offer patient education and support throughout the lung cancer treatment process.

Respiratory Therapist	Professionals who assess lung function, administer respiratory treatments, and provide education on breathing exercises and techniques to improve lung capacity and manage respiratory symptoms in lung cancer patients.
Genetic Counselor	Specialized in genetic counseling for patients and their families. They assess the risk of hereditary cancer syndromes, provide genetic testing, and offer guidance on cancer screening, prevention, and management options based on genetic information.
Interventional Radiologist	Specialists who use imaging techniques like CT scans or ultrasound to guide minimally invasive procedures for diagnosis or treatment. In the context of lung cancer, they may perform image-guided biopsies or place catheters for targeted delivery of therapies directly to the tumor site.
Pathologist	Medical doctors who examine lung tissue samples to diagnose lung cancer and determine its characteristics.

	They play a crucial role in identifying the type and stage of lung cancer, which helps guide treatment decisions and develop personalized care plans.
Registered Dietitian	Registered dietitians specialize in nutrition and provide guidance on healthy eating during lung cancer treatment. They assess nutritional needs, develop individualized meal plans, and address side effects that may affect diet. Dietitians help optimize nutrition to support the patient's overall health and well-being.
Social Worker	Social workers provide emotional support, counseling, and assistance with practical matters such as coordinating community resources, financial aid, and transportation. They help patients and their families navigate the challenges and complexities associated with lung cancer treatment and survivorship.
Psychologist or Psychiatrist	Psychologists or psychiatrists provide mental health support to lung cancer

	patients, addressing emotional and psychological aspects of their well-being. They offer counseling, therapy, and support to help patients cope with the challenges and stressors associated with lung cancer diagnosis, treatment, and survivorship.
Physical Therapist	Physical therapists focus on restoring and improving physical function, mobility, and overall well-being. They help lung cancer patients manage treatment-related side effects, improve strength and endurance, and enhance quality of life through targeted exercise, manual therapy, and education on self-care techniques.

Example: Breast Cancer Treatment Team at MD Anderson Cancer Center

The breast cancer treatment team at MD Anderson Cancer Center may include the following healthcare professionals shown in the table below.

Healthcare Professional	Description
Medical Oncologist	Specializes in medical oncology and focuses on breast cancer treatment.

	They develop personalized treatment plans, including chemotherapy, targeted therapy, or immunotherapy, and monitor the patient's response to treatment. They collaborate with other specialists to ensure comprehensive care.
Surgical Oncologist	Expert in performing surgical procedures for breast cancer, such as lumpectomy, mastectomy, or lymph node dissection. They assess the patient's surgical eligibility, perform the procedure, and work closely with the multidisciplinary team to provide optimal surgical outcomes and coordinate further treatment.
Radiation Oncologist	Specializes in radiation therapy for breast cancer. They utilize advanced techniques like intensity-modulated radiation therapy (IMRT) or brachytherapy to deliver precise radiation to the breast while minimizing exposure to healthy tissues, ensuring the best possible treatment outcomes.
Plastic Surgeon	Specializes in breast

	reconstruction surgery following mastectomy or lumpectomy. They collaborate with the surgical oncologist to provide patients with options for breast reconstruction and focus on restoring a natural appearance and enhancing quality of life.
Pathologist	Specializes in breast cancer pathology. They examine breast tissue samples, perform diagnostic tests, and provide detailed reports on the type, grade, and molecular characteristics of the cancer. This information helps guide treatment decisions and develop personalized care plans.
Radiologist	Specializes in breast imaging and interpretation of mammograms, ultrasounds, and breast MRI scans. They play a crucial role in detecting and characterizing breast abnormalities, aiding in diagnosis, treatment planning, and monitoring treatment response in breast cancer patients.
Nurse Navigator	A dedicated nurse who

	serves as a patient advocate and provides guidance and support throughout the breast cancer treatment journey. They assist patients in navigating appointments, coordinating care, and accessing support services, ensuring continuity and personalized care.
Genetic Counselor	Specializes in genetic counseling for breast cancer patients. They assess patients' genetic risk, provide counseling and testing options, and offer guidance on cancer prevention, screening, and management strategies based on inherited genetic factors.
Oncology Nurse	Registered nurses with expertise in breast cancer care. They provide direct patient care, administer medications, educate patients on treatment and side effects, and offer emotional support throughout the breast cancer treatment journey.
Social Worker	Licensed clinical social workers specializing in oncology. They provide emotional support and

	counseling to breast cancer patients, helping them cope with the psychological and social impact of their diagnosis. They also connect patients with resources and address practical and financial concerns.
Physical Therapist	Specializes in physical therapy for breast cancer patients. They focus on restoring physical function, improving mobility, managing treatment-related side effects, and enhancing quality of life through targeted exercise, manual therapy, and education on self-care techniques.
Registered Dietitian	Registered dietitians specializing in oncology nutrition. They assess patients' nutritional needs, develop individualized meal plans, and address side effects that may affect diet. Dietitians help optimize nutrition to support overall health and well-being during breast cancer treatment.
Psychologist or Psychiatrist	Specializes in providing mental health support to breast cancer patients,

	addressing emotional and psychological aspects of their well-being. They offer counseling, therapy, and support to help patients cope with the challenges and stressors associated with breast cancer diagnosis, treatment, and survivorship.
Nurse Practitioner	Advanced practice nurses with specialized training in oncology. They provide comprehensive care to breast cancer patients, including performing physical exams, ordering and interpreting diagnostic tests, prescribing medications, and educating patients on treatment options and management of side effects.
Palliative Care Specialist	Specializes in palliative care, focusing on improving the quality of life for breast cancer patients. They address symptom management, pain relief, and provide support to patients and their families throughout the treatment process.

Example: Colon Cancer Treatment Team at Johns Hopkins Hospital

The colon cancer treatment team at Johns Hopkins Hospital may include the following healthcare professionals shown in the table below.

Healthcare Professional	Description
Medical Oncologist	Specializes in medical oncology and focuses on colon cancer treatment. They develop personalized treatment plans, including chemotherapy, targeted therapy, or immunotherapy, and monitor the patient's response to treatment. They collaborate with other specialists to ensure comprehensive care.
Surgical Oncologist	Expert in performing surgical procedures for colon cancer, such as colectomy, polypectomy, or lymph node dissection. They assess the patient's surgical eligibility, perform the procedure, and work closely with the multidisciplinary team to provide optimal surgical outcomes and coordinate further treatment.
Radiation Oncologist	Specializes in radiation therapy for colon cancer. They utilize advanced techniques like intensity-modulated radiation therapy (IMRT) or brachytherapy to deliver precise radiation to

	the colon while minimizing exposure to healthy tissues, ensuring the best possible treatment outcomes.
Gastroenterologist	Specializes in the diagnosis and treatment of digestive system disorders, including colon cancer. They perform colonoscopies, biopsies, and other diagnostic procedures to assess the extent of the cancer and provide guidance on treatment options and follow-up care.
Pathologist	Specializes in examining tissue samples obtained from biopsies or surgical resections. They perform diagnostic tests and provide detailed reports on the type, stage, and molecular characteristics of the colon cancer. This information helps guide treatment decisions and develop personalized care plans.
Radiologist	Specializes in imaging and interpretation of diagnostic tests such as CT scans, MRIs, and PET scans. They play a crucial role in detecting and characterizing colon abnormalities, aiding in diagnosis, treatment planning, and monitoring treatment response in colon cancer

	patients.
Nurse Navigator	A dedicated nurse who serves as a patient advocate and provides guidance and support throughout the colon cancer treatment journey. They assist patients in navigating appointments, coordinating care, and accessing support services, ensuring continuity and personalized care.
Genetic Counselor	Specializes in genetic counseling for colon cancer patients. They assess patients' genetic risk, provide counseling and testing options, and offer guidance on cancer prevention, screening, and management strategies based on inherited genetic factors.
Oncology Nurse	Registered nurses with expertise in colon cancer care. They provide direct patient care, administer medications, educate patients on treatment and side effects, and offer emotional support throughout the colon cancer treatment journey.
Social Worker	Licensed clinical social workers specializing in oncology. They provide emotional support and counseling to colon cancer

	patients, helping them cope with the psychological and social impact of their diagnosis. They also connect patients with resources and address practical and financial concerns.
Nutritionist or Dietitian	Registered dietitians specializing in oncology nutrition. They assess patients' nutritional needs, develop individualized meal plans, and address side effects that may affect diet. Dietitians help optimize nutrition to support overall health and well-being during colon cancer treatment.
Physical Therapist	Specializes in physical therapy for colon cancer patients. They focus on restoring physical function, improving mobility, managing treatment-related side effects, and enhancing quality of life through targeted exercise, manual therapy, and education on self-care techniques.
Pharmacist	Specializes in medications used in colon cancer treatment. They play a crucial role in medication management, ensuring proper drug selection, dosage, and monitoring for potential drug interactions or side effects.

> Pharmacists collaborate with the treatment team to optimize medication therapy.

Key Considerations when Choosing a Medical Oncologist and/or Surgical Oncologist

As mentioned earlier, a medical oncologist is a physician who specializes in the diagnosis and treatment of cancer using systemic therapies such as chemotherapy, targeted therapy, immunotherapy, and hormonal therapy. They play a vital role in managing the medical aspects of a patient's cancer care, coordinating treatment plans, and monitoring their response to therapy.

To become a medical oncologist, extensive training is required. After completing medical school and obtaining a medical degree (MD or DO), individuals undergo a residency program in internal medicine, typically lasting three years. Following residency, they pursue a fellowship in medical oncology, which lasts two to three years. During this fellowship, they receive specialized training in oncology, including learning about different cancer types, treatment modalities, and conducting clinical research. After completing their fellowship, they may choose to pursue additional subspecialty training in a specific area of oncology.

When selecting a medical oncologist, several key considerations can help guide the decision-making process. These considerations include the oncologist's experience and expertise in treating the specific type and stage of cancer, their access to clinical trials and innovative treatments, their communication style and ability to provide comprehensive patient education, the reputation and quality of the medical institution or cancer center they are affiliated with, their availability and ability to provide personalized and timely care, and the compatibility and trust between the patient and the oncologist. Taking these factors into account can help ensure that patients receive optimal care and have a positive treatment experience.

Here's a table outlining key considerations when selecting a medical oncologist:

Consideration	Description
Specialty and Expertise	Assess the oncologist's experience and expertise in treating the specific type and stage of cancer you have. Consider whether they have treated similar cases and their familiarity with the latest advancements in cancer treatment.
Access to Clinical Trials	Determine if the oncologist has access to clinical trials and whether they actively participate in research. Clinical trials provide access to new treatments and can be an important consideration for patients seeking innovative therapies or options beyond standard treatments.
Communication and Education	Evaluate the

	oncologist's communication style and ability to provide comprehensive patient education. A good oncologist should be able to clearly explain the diagnosis, treatment options, potential side effects, and prognosis, and should be willing to answer questions and address concerns throughout the treatment journey.
Affiliation and Reputation	Consider the reputation and quality of the medical institution or cancer center where the oncologist practices. Look for centers with a multidisciplinary approach, access to supportive care services, and a strong track record in cancer care and research.
Availability and Accessibility	Assess the oncologist's availability and accessibility, including factors such as office location, appointment availability, and response time to

	inquiries. Consider whether they are accessible in case of emergencies or urgent concerns.
Patient-Oncologist Compatibility	Pay attention to the rapport and trust between the patient and the oncologist. Establishing a good relationship with the oncologist is important as it can positively impact the patient's overall experience and adherence to treatment.

A surgical oncologist or cancer surgeon is a specialized surgeon who focuses on the surgical treatment of cancer. They have expertise in performing surgical procedures to remove cancerous tumors, assess and stage the cancer, and manage surgical aspects of cancer care. Surgical oncologists work closely with the rest of the cancer treatment team to provide comprehensive and multidisciplinary care to patients.

To become a surgical oncologist, individuals first complete medical school and obtain a medical degree (MD or DO). Following medical school, they undergo a surgical residency program, typically lasting five to six years, to gain a solid foundation in general surgery. After completing their residency, they pursue additional fellowship in surgical oncology, which focuses on training specifically in the surgical management of cancer. During this fellowship, they gain expertise in various cancer types, advanced surgical techniques, and approaches to optimize oncologic outcomes while preserving organ function and quality of life.

When selecting a surgical oncologist, several key considerations can help guide the decision-making process. These considerations include the surgical oncologist's experience and expertise in treating the specific type of cancer, their surgical volume and outcomes, their familiarity with the latest surgical techniques and advancements, their affiliation with a reputable cancer center or hospital, their ability to work collaboratively with other members of the cancer treatment team, and their communication style and ability to provide comprehensive preoperative and postoperative care.

Here's a table outlining key considerations when selecting a surgical oncologist, along with surgical procedure thresholds for lung, breast, colon, pancreatic, and prostate cancer.

Consideration	Description	Procedure Threshold (approximate)
Specialty and Expertise	Assess the surgical oncologist's experience and expertise in treating the specific type of cancer you have. Consider their training, board certifications, and the number of years they have been practicing in the field of surgical oncology.	

Surgical Volume and Outcomes	Evaluate the surgeon's surgical volume and outcomes for the specific cancer type. Higher surgical volume is often associated with better outcomes. Consider their experience in performing complex surgeries, such as minimally invasive procedures or those requiring specialized techniques.	Lung: >20-30 lung cancer surgeries per year; Breast: >50 breast cancer surgeries per year; Colon: >20 colon cancer surgeries per year; Pancreatic: >10-15 pancreatic cancer surgeries per year; Prostate: >10-20 prostate cancer surgeries per year
Familiarity with Advanced Techniques	Determine if the surgical oncologist is familiar with the latest surgical techniques and advancements in the field. These may include minimally invasive procedures, robotic surgery, or other innovative approaches that can potentially offer benefits such as reduced pain, shorter hospital stays, and faster	

	recovery.
Affiliation and Reputation	Consider the affiliation of the surgical oncologist with a reputable cancer center or hospital. Look for centers known for their expertise in cancer care, multidisciplinary collaboration, access to clinical trials, and comprehensive support services.
Collaboration with Treatment Team	Assess the surgical oncologist's ability to work collaboratively with other members of the cancer treatment team, such as medical oncologists, radiation oncologists, and pathologists. A multidisciplinary approach is crucial for optimal treatment planning and coordination of care.
Communicatio	Evaluate the

n and Comprehensive Care	surgeon's communication style and their ability to provide comprehensive preoperative and postoperative care. A good surgical oncologist should explain the surgical procedure, potential risks and benefits, postoperative recovery, and provide ongoing support throughout the treatment journey.	

After you have narrowed down to a few doctors who are accepting new patients, set up appointments with them and ask them how much experience they have in treating your type of cancer, this question is extremely important, especially details such as what their success rate is, how do they define "success", how much they know about targeted therapy or immunotherapy. To find out if a doctor is board certified, you can obtain that information through the American Board of Medical Specialties (ABMS) at www.abms.org. The ABMS has a list of board-certified doctors who subscribe to the ABMS service. You can do a free search for all doctors in a certain specialty by state. Or you can type in the name of the doctor to learn about his (her) specialty. The American Society of Clinical Oncology (ASCO) provides a free, searchable database of ASCO member oncologists.

It's important to note that choosing a medical oncologist or a surgical oncologist is a personal decision, and it's important to find an oncologist who you feel comfortable with and who has the expertise and experience to treat your specific case. It's also important to consider the reputation and track record of the hospital or medical center where the oncologist practices.

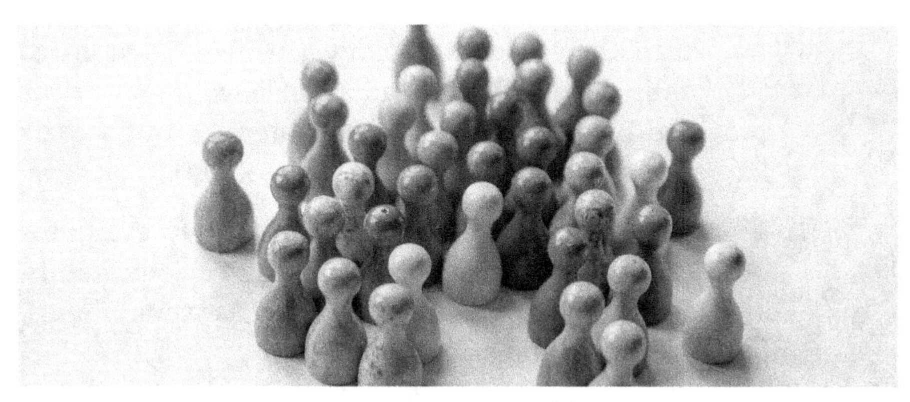

CHAPTER 16 TOP-RANKED US CANCER TREATMENT CENTERS

Several agencies rank cancer treatment centers in the United States based on various criteria. Some of the prominent agencies include:

1. U.S. News & World Report: U.S. News ranks cancer centers annually based on factors such as patient outcomes, specialized services, technologies, and reputation among physicians.

2. National Cancer Institute (NCI): NCI designates cancer centers as Comprehensive Cancer Centers, which signifies excellence in research, patient care, education, and community outreach. These centers are evaluated and selected based on rigorous criteria.

3. Commission on Cancer (CoC): CoC, a program of the American College of Surgeons, accredits cancer centers based on their compliance with quality standards, multidisciplinary care, research, and community outreach.

4. American College of Radiology (ACR): ACR assesses the quality and safety of radiation oncology services provided by cancer treatment centers through their Radiation Oncology Accreditation Program.

5. Leapfrog Group: Leapfrog Hospital Survey evaluates hospitals, including cancer centers, on various quality and safety measures, including patient outcomes, infection rates, and safety practices.

6. Centers for Medicare and Medicaid Services (CMS): CMS provides Hospital Compare data, which includes quality measures and patient satisfaction scores for cancer treatment centers participating in Medicare.

The ranking criteria of these agencies and their websites are shown in the table below

Agency	Ranking Criteria	Website
U.S. News & World Report	Patient outcomes, specialized services, technologies, reputation among physicians	https://health.usnews.com/best-hospitals
National Cancer Institute (NCI)	Excellence in research, patient care, education, community outreach	https://www.cancer.gov/research/nci-role/cancer-centers
Commission on Cancer (CoC)	Compliance with quality standards, multidisciplinary care, research, community outreach	https://www.facs.org/quality-programs/cancer
American College of Radiology (ACR)	Quality and safety of radiation oncology services	https://www.acr.org/Quality-Safety/Accreditation
Leapfrog Group	Quality and safety measures, patient outcomes, infection rates, safety practices	https://www.leapfroggroup.org/
Centers for Medicare and Medicaid Services (CMS)	Quality measures, patient satisfaction scores for Medicare participating cancer centers	https://www.medicare.gov/hospitalcompare

NCI-designated Comprehensive Cancer Centers

The National Cancer Institute (NCI) is part of the US National

Institutes for Health, and the NCI is dedicated to better understanding, diagnosing, treating, and preventing cancer. The NCI works with 71 cancer centers in the United States. It recognizes 3 levels of cancer treatment centers, ranging from a comprehensive cancer center to the more basic cancer treatment center. There are 54 cancer centers designated by NCI as Comprehensive Cancer Centers, which represent the highest level of recognition for excellence in cancer research, patient care, education, and community outreach.

The 54 Comprehensive Cancer Centers designated by the NCI are renowned for their exceptional contributions to cancer research, clinical trials, and the advancement of cancer care. These centers have demonstrated a commitment to conducting innovative laboratory research, translating scientific discoveries into clinical practice, and providing comprehensive and multidisciplinary care to cancer patients.

Each Comprehensive Cancer Center has a unique focus and expertise in various aspects of cancer research and treatment. These centers often have specialized programs and facilities dedicated to specific cancer types or research areas. They serve as major hubs for cutting-edge research, attracting top scientists, clinicians, and researchers who collaborate to drive advancements in cancer prevention, diagnosis, treatment, and survivorship.

The NCI-designated Comprehensive Cancer Centers also play a vital role in fostering collaborations and partnerships among academic institutions, healthcare providers, and the community. They contribute to cancer education and outreach programs, provide training opportunities for future cancer researchers and healthcare professionals, and actively engage with the local and national communities to raise awareness about cancer prevention and early detection.

Overall, the Comprehensive Cancer Centers designated by the NCI represent leaders in the field of cancer care and research, continuously striving to improve outcomes for cancer patients through innovative treatments, clinical trials, and community engagement.

A list of 19 Comprehensive Cancer Centers in major metropolitan area are shown in the table below

Comprehensive Cancer Center	City, State	Website
UCSF Helen Diller Family Comprehensive Cancer Center	San Francisco, CA	https://cancer.ucsf.edu/
UCLA Jonsson Comprehensive Cancer Center	Los Angeles, CA	https://www.cancer.ucla.edu/
Stanford Cancer Institute	Stanford, CA	https://med.stanford.edu/cancer.html
UC Davis Comprehensive Cancer Center	Sacramento, CA	https://health.ucdavis.edu/cancer/
UC San Diego Moores Cancer Center	La Jolla, CA	https://health.ucsd.edu/specialties/cancer/moores
MD Anderson Cancer Center	Houston, TX	https://www.mdanderson.org/
UT Southwestern Simmons Comprehensive Cancer Center	Dallas, TX	https://www.utsouthwestern.edu/
Memorial Sloan Kettering Cancer Center	New York, NY	https://www.mskcc.org/

Herbert Irving Comprehensive Cancer Center at Columbia University	New York, NY	https://www.hiccc.columbia.edu/
Dana-Farber/Brigham and Women's Cancer Center	Boston, MA	https://www.dana-farber.org/
Sidney Kimmel Comprehensive Cancer Center at Johns Hopkins	Baltimore, MD	https://www.hopkinsmedicine.org/kimmel_cancer_center/
Georgetown Lombardi Comprehensive Cancer Center	Washington, D.C.	https://lombardi.georgetown.edu/
Fred Hutchinson Cancer Research Center	Seattle, WA	https://www.fredhutch.org/
Moffitt Cancer Center	Tampa, FL	https://moffitt.org/
Sylvester Comprehensive Cancer Center	Miami, FL	https://umiamihealth.org/sylvester-comprehensive
UNC Lineberger Comprehensive Cancer Center	Chapel Hill, NC	https://unclineberger.org/
Robert H. Lurie Comprehensive Cancer Center	Chicago, IL	https://www.cancer.northwestern.edu/
The Ohio State University Comprehensive Cancer Center	Columbus, OH	https://cancer.osu.edu/

University of Colorado Cancer Center	Aurora, CO	https:// medschool.cuanschutz.edu/colorado-cancer-center

Top Cancer Centers Ranked by US News & World Report

A more well-known and highly reputable cancer center rankings is the one offered by U.S. News & World Report. First and foremost, U.S. News & World Report is a well-established and respected publication known for its comprehensive and rigorous approach to evaluating institutions across various fields, including healthcare. Their rankings are based on a thorough assessment of multiple factors, including patient outcomes, research activities, expertise of healthcare professionals, advanced technologies, and patient services.

U.S. News & World Report employs a robust methodology that involves analyzing objective data, such as survival rates, patient safety measures, and the volume of complex procedures performed. They also conduct surveys of medical professionals to gather subjective input regarding the reputation and quality of cancer centers. This combination of objective and subjective assessments provides a comprehensive evaluation of the cancer centers' overall performance.

Moreover, the rankings are updated annually, ensuring that the information is current and reflective of the latest advancements and achievements in cancer care. The transparency of the methodology and the detailed information provided by U.S. News & World Report allow patients and their families to make informed decisions when selecting a cancer center for their care.

Overall, the U.S. News & World Report cancer center rankings are widely recognized and trusted by patients, healthcare professionals, and the healthcare industry as a whole, making them a considerable and reputable resource for individuals seeking high-quality cancer treatment.

Let's take a look at the top 20 cancer treatment centers in the US respectively for lung cancer, breast cancer, colon cancer and prostate cancer.

Here is a table showing the top 20 lung cancer treatment centers in the US, their city location, and contact phone number based on the 2021-22 U.S. News & World Report rankings.

Rank	Lung Cancer Treatment Center	City	Phone Number
1	MD Anderson Cancer Center	Houston, TX	713-792-2121
2	Memorial Sloan Kettering Cancer Center	New York, NY	212-639-2000
3	Mayo Clinic	Rochester, MN	507-284-2511
4	Cleveland Clinic	Cleveland, OH	216-444-2200
5	Johns Hopkins Hospital	Baltimore, MD	410-955-5000
6	Dana-Farber/Brigham and Women's Cancer Center	Boston, MA	617-632-3000
7	Cedars-Sinai Medical Center	Los Angeles, CA	310-423-5000
8	Stanford Health Care	Stanford, CA	650-723-4000
9	University of California, San Francisco Medical Center	San Francisco, CA	415-476-1000
10	New York-Presbyterian Hospital-Columbia and Cornell	New York, NY	212-746-5454
11	Northwestern Memorial Hospital	Chicago, IL	312-926-2000

12	Ronald Reagan UCLA Medical Center	Los Angeles, CA	310-825-9111
13	Mount Sinai Hospital	New York, NY	212-241-6500
14	Barnes-Jewish Hospital	St. Louis, MO	314-747-3000
15	University of Michigan Hospitals-Michigan Medicine	Ann Arbor, MI	734-936-4000
16	Moffitt Cancer Center	Tampa, FL	813-745-4673
17	Huntsman Cancer Institute at the University of Utah	Salt Lake City, UT	801-585-0100
18	University of Colorado Hospital	Aurora, CO	720-848-0000
19	Roswell Park Comprehensive Cancer Center	Buffalo, NY	716-845-2300
20	Vanderbilt University Medical Center	Nashville, TN	615-322-5000

Here is a table showing the top 20 breast cancer treatment centers in the US, their city location, and contact phone number based on the 2021-22 U.S. News & World Report rankings.

Rank	Breast Cancer Treatment Center	City	Phone Number
1	Memorial Sloan Kettering Cancer Center	New York, NY	212-639-2000
2	MD Anderson Cancer Center	Houston, TX	713-792-2121
3	Mayo Clinic	Rochester, MN	507-284-2511
4	Dana-Farber/Brigham and Women's Cancer	Boston, MA	617-632-3000

	Center		
5	Johns Hopkins Hospital	Baltimore, MD	410-955-5000
6	Cleveland Clinic	Cleveland, OH	216-444-2200
7	Stanford Health Care	Stanford, CA	650-723-4000
8	University of California, San Francisco Medical Center	San Francisco, CA	415-476-1000
9	NewYork-Presbyterian Hospital-Columbia and Cornell	New York, NY	212-746-5454
10	Northwestern Memorial Hospital	Chicago, IL	312-926-2000
11	University of Michigan Hospitals-Michigan Medicine	Ann Arbor, MI	734-936-4000
12	Mount Sinai Hospital	New York, NY	212-241-6500
13	Ronald Reagan UCLA Medical Center	Los Angeles, CA	310-825-9111
14	Cedars-Sinai Medical Center	Los Angeles, CA	310-423-5000
15	Barnes-Jewish Hospital	St. Louis, MO	314-747-3000
16	Moffitt Cancer Center	Tampa, FL	813-745-4673
17	University of Colorado Hospital	Aurora, CO	720-848-0000
18	Roswell Park Comprehensive Cancer Center	Buffalo, NY	716-845-2300
19	Huntsman Cancer Institute at the University of Utah	Salt Lake City, UT	801-585-0100
20	Vanderbilt University	Nashville, TN	615-322-5000

Medical Center

Here is a table showing the top 20 colon cancer treatment centers in the US, their city location, and contact phone number based on the 2021-22 U.S. News & World Report rankings.

Rank	Colon Cancer Treatment Center	City	Phone Number
1	MD Anderson Cancer Center	Houston, TX	713-792-2121
2	Memorial Sloan Kettering Cancer Center	New York, NY	212-639-2000
3	Mayo Clinic	Rochester, MN	507-284-2511
4	Cleveland Clinic	Cleveland, OH	216-444-2200
5	Johns Hopkins Hospital	Baltimore, MD	410-955-5000
6	Dana-Farber/Brigham and Women's Cancer Center	Boston, MA	617-632-3000
7	Cedars-Sinai Medical Center	Los Angeles, CA	310-423-5000
8	Stanford Health Care	Stanford, CA	650-723-4000
9	University of California, San Francisco Medical Center	San Francisco, CA	415-476-1000
10	New York-Presbyterian Hospital-Columbia and Cornell	New York, NY	212-746-5454
11	Northwestern Memorial Hospital	Chicago, IL	312-926-2000
12	Ronald Reagan UCLA Medical Center	Los Angeles, CA	310-825-9111

13	Mount Sinai Hospital	New York, NY	212-241-6500
14	Barnes-Jewish Hospital	St. Louis, MO	314-747-3000
15	University of Michigan Hospitals-Michigan Medicine	Ann Arbor, MI	734-936-4000
16	Moffitt Cancer Center	Tampa, FL	813-745-4673
17	Huntsman Cancer Institute at the University of Utah	Salt Lake City, UT	801-585-0100
18	University of Colorado Hospital	Aurora, CO	720-848-0000
19	Roswell Park Comprehensive Cancer Center	Buffalo, NY	716-845-2300
20	Vanderbilt University Medical Center	Nashville, TN	615-322-5000

Here is a table showing the top 20 prostate cancer treatment centers in the US, their city location, and contact phone number based on the 2021-22 U.S. News & World Report rankings.

Rank	Prostate Cancer Treatment Center	City	Phone Number
1	Mayo Clinic	Rochester, MN	507-284-2511
2	Cleveland Clinic	Cleveland, OH	216-444-2200
3	Johns Hopkins Hospital	Baltimore, MD	410-955-5000
4	Memorial Sloan Kettering Cancer Center	New York, NY	212-639-2000
5	MD Anderson Cancer Center	Houston, TX	713-792-2121
6	New York-Presbyterian	New York, NY	212-746-5454

	Hospital-Columbia and Cornell		
7	UCLA Medical Center	Los Angeles, CA	310-825-9111
8	Cedars-Sinai Medical Center	Los Angeles, CA	310-423-5000
9	University of California, San Francisco Medical Center	San Francisco, CA	415-476-1000
10	Dana-Farber/Brigham and Women's Cancer Center	Boston, MA	617-632-3000
11	University of Michigan Hospitals-Michigan Medicine	Ann Arbor, MI	734-936-4000
12	Northwestern Memorial Hospital	Chicago, IL	312-926-2000
13	Stanford Health Care	Stanford, CA	650-723-4000
14	Barnes-Jewish Hospital	St. Louis, MO	314-747-3000
15	University of Colorado Hospital	Aurora, CO	720-848-0000
16	Moffitt Cancer Center	Tampa, FL	813-745-4673
17	H. Lee Moffitt Cancer Center and Research Institute	Tampa, FL	888-663-3488
18	Roswell Park Comprehensive Cancer Center	Buffalo, NY	716-845-2300
19	Huntsman Cancer Institute at the University of Utah	Salt Lake City, UT	801-585-0100
20	Vanderbilt University	Nashville, TN	615-322-5000

Medical Center

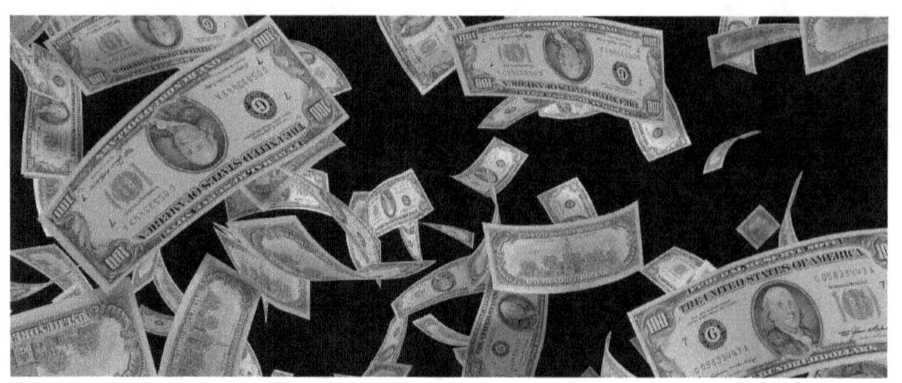

SECTION V MANAGING CANCER TREATMENT COSTS

Cancer is a costly disease for a number of reasons. First and foremost, the treatments for cancer are often complex and can involve a range of procedures, including surgeries, radiation therapy, chemotherapy, targeted therapy, and immunotherapy. These treatments are typically expensive, and the cost can vary depending on the type and stage of cancer, the type of treatment, and the duration of treatment.

Here is a table showing the approximate cost per month for some commonly used cancer drugs for chemotherapy, targeted therapy, and immunotherapy:

Drug Name	Type	Annual Cost (USD)
Keytruda	Immunotherapy	$150,000 - $200,000
Opdivo	Immunotherapy	$150,000 - $200,000

Yervoy	Immunotherapy	$250,000 - $300,000
Kymriah	Immunotherapy	$373,000
Imfinzi	Immunotherapy	$180,000
Tecentriq	Immunotherapy	$150,000 - $200,000
Avastin	Targeted Therapy	$100,000 - $120,000
Herceptin	Targeted Therapy	$70,000 - $80,000
Gleevec	Targeted Therapy	$146,000 - $172,000
Tagrisso	Targeted Therapy	$179,200
Tarceva	Targeted Therapy	$92,000 - $94,000
Abraxane	Chemotherapy	$109,000
FOLFOX	Chemotherapy	$35,000
Taxol	Chemotherapy	$8,000
Doxorubicin	Chemotherapy	$12,000

In addition to the cost of treatment, there are a number of other factors that can contribute to the cost of cancer care. For example, patients with cancer may require additional medical care, such as follow-up appointments, laboratory tests, and imaging studies. They may also require supportive care, such as pain management, nutrition support, and psychological counseling. These services can add to the overall cost of care.

Moreover, cancer can result in indirect costs, such as lost productivity due to time off work, travel expenses associated with treatment, and the need for care-giving assistance. In some cases, patients may also face financial hardship due to the cost of cancer care, which can lead to significant stress and anxiety.

Examples of dollar values for cancer treatment in recent years are staggering. According to a report published by the American Society of Clinical Oncology in 2020, the cost of cancer care in the United States is estimated to be $156 billion annually. A study published in the Journal of the National Cancer Institute estimated that the average cost of treating metastatic breast cancer in the first year of diagnosis was approximately $134,000 in 2015. Another study published in the Journal of Clinical Oncology estimated that the median cost of treating advanced lung cancer with immunotherapy was approximately $250,000 in 2019.

Overall, cancer is a costly disease due to the complexity of its treatments, the need for supportive care, and the potential for indirect costs. The high cost of cancer care can have significant financial implications for patients and their families, and it highlights the need for strategies to manage costs and improve access to care.

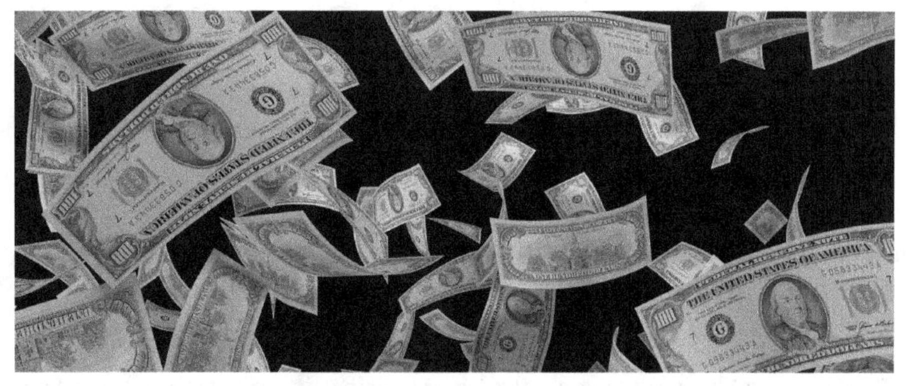

CHAPTER 17 CANCER CARE
WITH PRIVATE INSURANCE,
OBAMACARE AND MEDICARE

Managing the cost of cancer treatment can be a daunting task for patients and their families. With the high cost of cancer care, it's essential to have a plan in place to manage these expenses. In this chapter, we will discuss how to manage the cost of cancer treatment with private insurance, Obamacare, and Medicare.

Private Insurance

Private insurance plans vary widely in terms of coverage and limitations for cancer treatment. However, most private insurance plans cover cancer treatment to some extent, although the amount of coverage and out-of-pocket costs can vary significantly.

Private insurance plans typically cover standard cancer treatments, such as chemotherapy, radiation therapy, and surgery. However, some plans may have restrictions on certain treatments, such as experimental therapies or alternative treatments.

In terms of costs, most private insurance plans require patients to pay a portion of the costs through copayments, deductibles, and coinsurance. These out-of-pocket costs can be significant, especially for high-cost treatments. Additionally, some plans may have annual or lifetime caps on coverage for cancer treatment, which can leave patients with significant medical bills.

To manage the cost of cancer treatment with private insurance, patients should review their insurance policies carefully to understand their coverage and out-of-pocket costs. It is also important to communicate with the insurance company and healthcare providers to negotiate discounts and payment plans. Some private insurance plans may offer programs to help patients manage the cost of cancer treatment, such as patient assistance programs or financial counseling.

Here are some tips on how to manage the cost of cancer treatment with private insurance:

1. Review your insurance plan: It's important to understand what your insurance plan covers and what it does not cover. Review your insurance plan's policy and understand your out-of-pocket costs.

2. Choose in-network providers: Choosing in-network providers can save you money on your medical bills. If you go out-of-network, your insurance company may not cover the cost of your treatment, or you may have to pay a higher deductible.

3. Ask for pre-authorization: Before receiving any medical treatment, ask your insurance company if pre-authorization is required. Pre-authorization is a process where the insurance company approves the medical treatment before it is provided. This can help avoid unexpected medical bills.

4. Negotiate costs: Talk to your healthcare provider about the

cost of your treatment. You may be able to negotiate a lower cost or a payment plan that works for you.

5. Look for financial assistance programs: Many pharmaceutical companies offer financial assistance programs for their medications. Additionally, there are several nonprofit organizations that provide financial assistance to cancer patients. Research these programs and see if you qualify.

Obamacare

Obamacare, also known as the Affordable Care Act (ACA), was implemented in 2010 to increase the availability of affordable health insurance and to improve the quality of healthcare. Under Obamacare, cancer treatment is covered as an essential health benefit. This means that health insurance plans must cover cancer treatment services, including chemotherapy, radiation therapy, surgery, and follow-up care.

Obamacare has certain limitations when it comes to cancer treatment coverage. For example, while insurance plans must cover cancer treatment, the amount of coverage provided may vary depending on the specific plan. Some plans may require patients to pay out-of-pocket costs, such as deductibles, copays, and coinsurance, which can be expensive. Additionally, some cancer treatments, such as experimental therapies or certain prescription drugs, may not be covered by all insurance plans.

However, Obamacare does provide some protections for cancer patients. For example, insurance companies cannot deny coverage to individuals with pre-existing conditions, including cancer. Additionally, Obamacare includes cost-sharing reductions for low-income individuals, which can help reduce out-of-pocket costs for cancer treatment.

Medicare

Medicare is a federal health insurance program that provides coverage to eligible individuals who are 65 years or older, individuals with certain disabilities, and individuals with end-stage renal disease. Medicare covers cancer treatment, including chemotherapy, radiation therapy, and surgical procedures, as well as some medications used to treat cancer. However, Medicare has limitations and out-of-pocket costs for cancer patients.

Medicare Part A covers inpatient hospital stays, skilled nursing facility stays, and hospice care. Part A typically covers the costs of chemotherapy and radiation therapy received as an inpatient in a hospital. Medicare Part B covers medically necessary outpatient services and preventive services, including doctor visits, laboratory tests, and diagnostic imaging. Part B covers chemotherapy and radiation therapy received as an outpatient at a hospital or doctor's office. Medicare Part D covers prescription drugs, including oral chemotherapy and targeted therapy drugs.

However, Medicare has some limitations and out-of-pocket costs for cancer patients. Part A has a deductible for hospital stays, and Part B has a deductible and coinsurance for outpatient services. Part D has a monthly premium, deductible, and coinsurance for prescription drugs. There is also a coverage gap or "donut hole" in Part D, where patients pay a higher percentage of their prescription drug costs until they reach catastrophic coverage.

Additionally, Medicare does not cover certain types of cancer treatment, such as some experimental treatments or treatments that are not deemed medically necessary. Cancer patients may also face additional costs, such as transportation, parking, and lodging for treatment, which are not covered by Medicare.

Overall, while Medicare covers a range of cancer treatments and medications, cancer patients may still face significant out-of-pocket costs and limitations. It is important for cancer patients to carefully review their Medicare coverage and consider supplemental insurance or financial assistance programs to help manage their treatment costs.

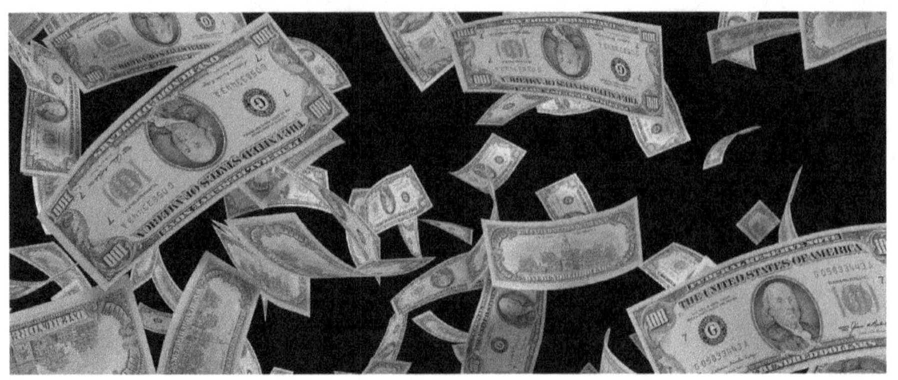

CHAPTER 18 STRATEGIES TO SAVE MONEY ON CANCER CARE

There are several options available for cancer patients to manage their treatment costs more effectively and even save money. The first and foremost option is to seek a second opinion from a top cancer center, as approximately 10% of cancer patients receive a misdiagnosis, especially if the initial diagnosis was done in a rural medical facility. A second opinion can confirm the original diagnosis, or it may reveal a different type or stage of cancer, which will lead to changes in the treatment plan. Additionally, a second opinion may offer additional treatment options for the patient to consider. The good news is that most insurance plans cover second opinions for surgery or other major medical procedures, although prescription coverage may vary. Therefore, it is advisable to check with the insurance provider for approval before proceeding with a second opinion.

Another option is to review medical insurance policies before beginning treatment and consult with the employee benefits administrator to understand the coverage limitations and out-of-pocket costs. Some cancer patients have policies with a $200,000 or $500,000 lifetime maximum, which can be exhausted quickly. Therefore, patients should consider these numbers before starting treatment and negotiate discounts off certain medical charges with their provider to preserve their lifetime maximum.

All health insurance carriers are required to provide their members with a Summary Plan Description that contains information about specific coverage benefits. Cancer patients should read this document carefully and examine all explanations of benefits statements and other insurance documents they receive. If they find it challenging to understand these documents, they should reach out to the insurance provider, hospital, or patient advocate group for help.

Foundations and Charitable organizations

Foundations and charitable organizations play an important role in supporting cancer patients and cancer treatment in various ways. These organizations may provide financial assistance, educational resources, emotional support, and advocacy for cancer patients and their families.

1) Financial Assistance: Many foundations and organizations provide financial assistance to cancer patients to help with the cost of treatment, medications, transportation, and other related expenses. This can be especially helpful for those who are underinsured or have limited financial resources.

2) Educational Resources: Some organizations provide educational resources and information about cancer, treatment options, and support services. These resources can help patients make informed decisions about their care and provide them with the tools they need to manage their condition.

3) Emotional Support: Living with cancer can be emotionally challenging for patients and their families. Charitable organizations often provide counseling services, support groups, and other forms of emotional support to help patients cope with the stress and anxiety of a cancer diagnosis.

4) Advocacy: Many organizations also advocate for cancer patients by raising awareness about the disease and advocating for better access to treatment, research, and support services. They may also work to change policies and laws to improve cancer care and quality of life for patients and their families.

Overall, foundations and charitable organizations play a vital role in helping cancer patients access the care and support they need to manage their condition and improve their quality of life.

Below a table with foundations for cancer patients with lung cancer, breast cancer, colon cancer, prostate cancer, and pancreatic cancer, along with their phone numbers and website addresses.

Cancer Type	Foundation	Phone Number	Website
Lung Cancer	LUNGevity Foundation	312-464-0716	www.lungevity.org
Lung Cancer	Bonnie J. Addario Lung Cancer Foundation	650-598-2857	www.lungcancerfoundation.org
Lung Cancer	Lung Cancer Research Foundation	212-448-0700	https://www.lungcancerresearchfoundation.org/
Breast Cancer	Susan G. Komen Breast Cancer Foundation	877-465-6636	www.komen.org
Breast Cancer	Breast Cancer Research Foundation	646-497-2600	www.bcrf.org
Colon Cancer	Colorectal Cancer Alliance	877-422-2030	www.ccalliance.org
Colon Cancer	Colon Cancer Foundation	914-305-6674	https://coloncancerfoundation.org/
Colon Cancer	Fight Colorectal Cancer	877-427-2111	www.fightcrc.org
Prostate Cancer	Prostate Cancer Foundation	310-570-4700	www.pcf.org
Prostate Cancer	ZERO - The End of Prostate Cancer	844-244-1309	www.zerocancer.org
Pancreatic Cancer	Pancreatic Cancer Action Network	877-272-6226	www.pancan.org
Pancreatic Cancer	Lustgarten Foundation	866-789-1000	www.lustgarten.org

The Patient Advocate Foundation (PAF) is a non-profit organization that provides case management services to people with chronic, debilitating, or life-threatening illnesses. They help patients understand their insurance coverage and anticipate potential medical expenses. Patients are encouraged to call their case managers at any point in their diagnosis for assistance at no cost. PAF actively works to connect patients with a suitable organization or service that can help. Moreover, they offer a Co-Pay Relief Program to assist patients in managing pharmaceutical co-payments through mail-order prescriptions, state and federal funds, or prescription drug cards.

Similarly, some cancer centers and hospitals offer their own Financial Hardship and Travel Assistance Programs to help patients. For those who do not qualify for travel assistance programs, there are a number of air travel companies that offer free or reduced-fare transportation services. The Air Charity Network can help arrange flights for patients in all 50 states, and the Corporate Angel Network helps patients fly for free in empty seats on corporate jets. The US has several cancer patient assistance programs available, as listed in the table below.

Organization	Description	Phone Number	Website
Patient Advocate Foundation	Provides case management services to people with chronic, debilitating, or life-threatening illnesses. Offers Co-Pay Relief Program to help manage pharmaceutical co-payments.	800-532-5274	https://www.patientadvocate.org/
CancerCare Co-Payment Assistance Foundation	Provides co-payment assistance for chemotherapy and targeted treatment drugs.	866-552-6729	https://www.cancercarecopay.org/
Healthwell Foundation	Provides financial assistance to cover out-of-pocket expenses for eligible individuals with insurance who are living with chronic or life-altering conditions.	800-675-8416	https://www.healthwellfoundation.org/
The Leukemia & Lymphoma Society	Offers financial assistance for patients with blood cancer.	888-557-7177	https://www.lls.org/support/financial-support
National Organization for Rare Disorders	Provides financial assistance for medications, insurance premiums, co-payments, and incidental medical expenses for patients with rare diseases.	800-999-6673	https://rarediseases.org/
Cancer Financial Assistance Coalition	A group of organizations that offer financial assistance to cancer patients.	866-55-CFAC	https://www.cancerfac.org/

Air Charity Network	Arranges free air transportation for patients in need.	877-621-7177	https://www.aircharitynetwork.org/
Corporate Angel Network	Arranges free air transportation for cancer patients in empty seats on corporate jets.	866-328-1313	https://www.corpangelnetwork.org/
Joe's House	A nonprofit organization that helps cancer patients and their families find lodging during treatment.	877-563-7468	https://www.joeshouse.org/
American Cancer Society	Provides lodging assistance and transportation assistance to cancer patients.	800-227-2345	https://www.cancer.org/

In case you are wondering, here's a success story of a cancer patient who received financial assistance from the American Cancer Society (ACS):

Jane was a 48-year-old mother of two who was diagnosed with breast cancer. She had health insurance through her employer, but her treatment was going to cost more than she could afford. She was worried about how she was going to pay for it all and still take care of her family.

A social worker at the hospital where Jane was receiving treatment suggested she reach out to the American Cancer Society for help. Jane was hesitant at first, but she decided to call the ACS hotline and was connected with a representative who explained the financial assistance programs available to her.

With the help of the ACS, Jane was able to apply for and receive a grant to help cover the cost of her treatment. She also received support from ACS volunteers who provided her with transportation to and from her appointments and emotional support during her journey.

Thanks to the financial assistance and support provided by the ACS, Jane was able to focus on her treatment and recovery without worrying about the financial burden it would place on her and her family.

GoFundMe is a popular crowdfunding platform that can be

used by cancer patients to raise funds for their treatment, as well as some social media channels. Another option for a cancer patient is to get supplemental lump-sum cancer insurance policy that provides a lump-sum cash payment of up to $100,000. The payment can be used for medical and non-medical bills. These insurance policies are offered at websites such as www.cancerinsurance.com. However, it is important to understand that these supplemental insurance policies are usually offered before one has been diagnosed with cancer. Thus, a cancer patient may be denied coverage.

It is important to note that before signing up for any insurance policy, one should carefully read the terms and conditions, including coverage limitations and exclusions. It is also advisable to consult with an insurance agent to understand the benefits and limitations of various policies before making a decision.

Enrolling in a Clinical Trial

Enrolling in a clinical trial can also be a viable option for cancer patients to receive treatment at a reduced cost, and in some cases, even free of charge. Clinical trials are research studies that test new treatments, therapies, or interventions for cancer. Participating in a clinical trial can provide access to treatments that are not yet available to the general public. A cancer patient can speak with the cancer treatment team to identify clinical trials that may be appropriate for his(her) condition, or search for clinical trials through resources such as ClinicalTrials.gov, a database of publicly and privately funded clinical studies conducted around the world. Additionally, many cancer centers and hospitals have their own clinical trial databases. The patient will need to undergo screening to meet the eligibility criteria for the study, which may include factors such as age, cancer type and stage and previous treatments etc. Once accepted through the clinical trial sponsor who is funding the study, the patient will need to follow the trial protocol closely, which may include attending regular appointments and receiving treatments as prescribed.

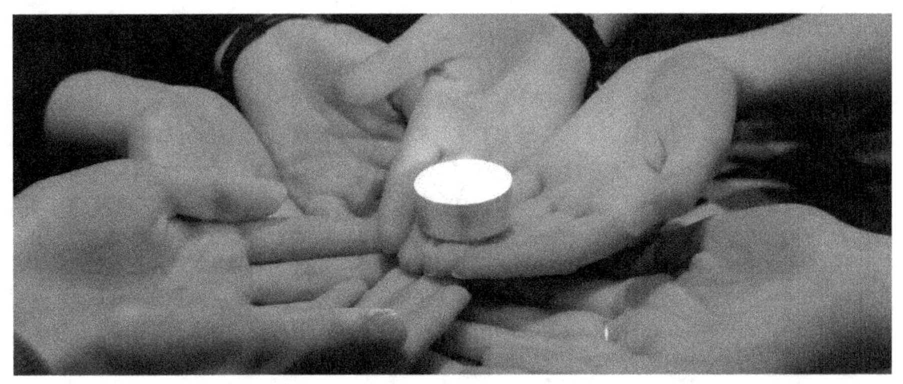

SECTION VI SUPPORTING CANCER PATIENTS AND SURVIVORS WITH PALLIATIVE CARE

More and more people after a cancer diagnosis are living fuller lives and surviving longer, yet there is a difference between a cancer patient and a cancer survivor. A cancer patient is someone who has been diagnosed with cancer and is currently undergoing treatment or monitoring to manage their cancer. Cancer patients may experience a range of physical and emotional challenges related to their diagnosis and treatment, including pain, fatigue, anxiety, and depression. They may need to make significant adjustments to their daily lives, such as taking time off work, changing their diet and exercise routines, and managing their side effects. A cancer survivor, on the other hand, is someone who has completed their cancer treatment, regardless of whether they are currently in remission or not. This term encompasses a wide range of individuals who have faced a life-threatening disease and have overcome significant physical, emotional, and psychological challenges. They may have undergone surgery, chemotherapy, radiation therapy, immunotherapy, or a combination of treatments to manage their cancer. Once treatment is complete, the survivor may continue to receive follow-up care and monitoring to detect any signs of cancer recurrence. Survivors may continue to experience physical and emotional effects related to their cancer and treatment, but they have transitioned to a different phase in their cancer journey. Survivors may also face challenges related to adjusting to life after cancer treatment, such as returning to work, managing ongoing health issues, and navigating their relationships with friends and family.

It is important to note that the terms "patient" and "survivor" are not mutually exclusive, as a cancer patient may also be a cancer survivor if they have completed treatment and are living beyond their cancer diagnosis. The number of cancer patients and survivors has increased significantly over the years due to advancements in cancer diagnosis and treatment. According to the American Cancer Society, there were an estimated 1.8 million new cancer cases diagnosed in the United States in 2020, and an estimated 16.9 million cancer survivors. The table below shows the estimated number of cancer patients and survivors in the United States by year:

Year	New Cancer Cases	Cancer Survivors
2020	1.8 million	16.9 million
2010	1.5 million	11.9 million
2000	1.2 million	8.0 million
1990	1.0 million	3.0 million

Cancer patients and survivors will likely face difficulties in their daily lives, including challenges at work and at home. Cancer treatment can be physically and emotionally draining, and patients may need to take time off work to manage their treatment and recovery. Survivors may also face ongoing health issues related to their cancer and treatment, which can include physical side effects such as fatigue, neuropathy, and chronic pain, as well as emotional and psychological challenges such as anxiety, depression, and fear of recurrence. These challenges can impact survivors' ability to work and fulfill their responsibilities at home, which can lead to financial and emotional stress.

Relationships with family members, friends, and the general public can also be impacted by a cancer diagnosis. Loved ones may struggle to understand the patient or survivor's experience and may unintentionally say or do things that are hurtful. The general public may also have misconceptions about cancer and cancer treatment, which can lead to stigma and discrimination, or may wrongly assume cancer survivors are no longer at risk for cancer or that they should be fully recovered.

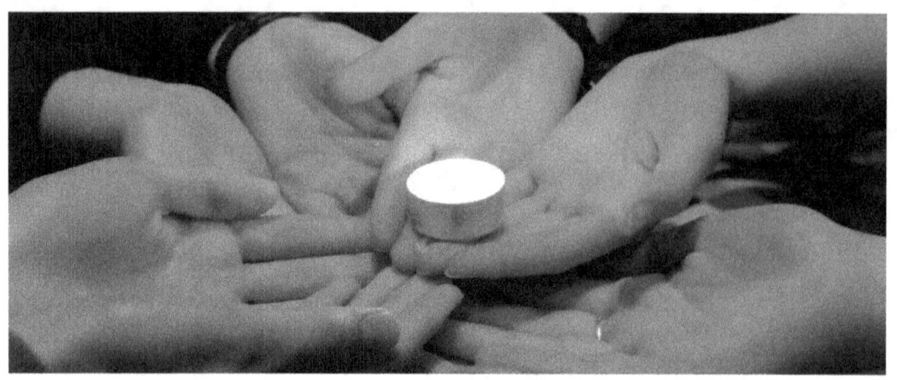

CHAPTER 19 UNDERSTANDING PALLIATIVE CARE

With the number of cancer patients and survivors increasing over the years, it is important to continue to raise awareness about the needs of cancer patients and survivors and provide support to help them manage their cancer journey.

Overall, cancer survivorship is a complex journey that requires ongoing support and resources. While the number of cancer survivors has increased over the years (is expected to increase to over 22 million by 2030), it is important to continue to raise awareness about survivorship issues and provide support to those who have overcome this life-threatening disease.

There are several organizations dedicated to supporting cancer survivors and their families, such as the American Cancer Society and the National Cancer Institute. These organizations provide a variety of resources, including support groups, educational materials, and financial assistance to help cancer survivors navigate the challenges they may face after treatment.

One powerful approach that can be used to enhance the quality of life for cancer patients, cancer survivors and their caregivers is palliative care. Palliative care for cancer patients is a specialized approach to medical care that focuses on improving the quality of life of individuals with cancer. The goal of palliative care is to provide relief from the symptoms, pain, and stress associated with cancer and its treatment, regardless of the stage of the disease.

Palliative care is not the same as hospice care, which is a type of end-of-life care provided to individuals who are nearing the end of their lives. Palliative care can be provided at any point during a cancer patient's journey, from the time of diagnosis through treatment and beyond. The American Society of Clinical Oncologists recommends that all patients with advanced cancer receive palliative care.

Palliative care for cancer patients may involve a multidisciplinary team of healthcare professionals, including physicians, nurses, social workers, and chaplains. The team works together to address the physical, emotional, and spiritual needs of the patient and their family.

The services provided by palliative care for cancer patients may include:

- Pain and symptom management: Palliative care providers work to manage the physical symptoms of cancer, such as pain, nausea, and fatigue.

- Emotional and spiritual support: Palliative care providers can help patients and their families cope with the emotional and spiritual challenges of cancer, such as anxiety, depression, and loss of meaning or purpose.

- Care coordination: Palliative care providers can work with the patient's other healthcare providers to ensure that their medical care is well-coordinated.

- Advanced care planning: Palliative care providers can assist patients and their families with making decisions about end-of-life care and other medical decisions.

- Family support: Palliative care providers can offer support to the patient's family members, including counseling, education, and referrals to other resources.

Overall, palliative care for cancer patients aims to improve the quality of life of individuals with cancer and their families, by addressing the physical, emotional, and spiritual aspects of their care. It can be an important component of cancer treatment, helping patients to manage their symptoms and improve their well-being.

Example: Palliative care for lung cancer patients

Lung cancer is a type of cancer that can be difficult to manage, as it often presents with significant symptoms such as coughing, shortness of breath, and chest pain. One of the challenges of palliative care for lung cancer patients is managing these symptoms to improve the patient's quality of life.

One specific intervention that can be used in palliative care for lung cancer patients is the use of oxygen therapy to improve breathing. Oxygen therapy involves providing the patient with a higher concentration of oxygen than is available in the air, which can help to alleviate symptoms.

Shortness of breath can be caused by the cancer itself, as well as by treatments such as chemotherapy and radiation therapy. One specific intervention that can be used in palliative care for lung cancer patients to address this challenge is pulmonary rehabilitation. Pulmonary rehabilitation is a program of exercises and education that can improve lung function and reduce shortness of breath. It can also help patients build endurance and strength and may include breathing techniques to help manage shortness of breath.

Pain is another common symptom of lung cancer and can be

caused by the cancer itself as well as by treatments. Palliative care providers can help manage pain by prescribing medications such as opioids or nonsteroidal anti-inflammatory drugs (NSAIDs). They may also recommend non-pharmacological interventions such as massage, acupuncture, or physical therapy to help manage pain.

Fatigue is also a common symptom of lung cancer that can be addressed through palliative care. Fatigue can be caused by the cancer itself, as well as by treatments such as chemotherapy and radiation therapy. Palliative care providers can recommend lifestyle modifications such as exercise or relaxation techniques to help manage fatigue. Addressing underlying factors such as anemia or sleep disorders may also help to reduce fatigue.

In addition to managing symptoms such as shortness of breath and pain, palliative care for lung cancer patients can also involve emotional and psychological support. Lung cancer can be a very stressful and difficult diagnosis for patients and their families, and palliative care providers can offer counseling and support to help patients and their families cope with the emotional and psychological effects of the disease.

Example: Palliative care for breast cancer patients

Breast cancer is a type of cancer that can present significant challenges for patients, including physical symptoms such as pain, fatigue, and nausea, as well as emotional and psychological challenges related to the diagnosis and treatment of the disease. One of the key challenges in palliative care for breast cancer patients is managing these symptoms to improve the patient's quality of life.

One specific intervention that can be used in palliative care for breast cancer patients is the use of pain medication to manage pain. Depending on the severity of the pain, doctors may prescribe opioids, nonsteroidal anti-inflammatory drugs (NSAIDs), or other pain medications. Patients may also be referred to physical therapy or other rehabilitation programs to help manage pain and improve physical function.

Fatigue is another common symptom of breast cancer that can significantly impact a patient's quality of life. Palliative care providers may recommend lifestyle modifications such as exercise or relaxation techniques to help manage fatigue. Additionally, addressing underlying factors such as anemia or sleep disorders may also help to reduce fatigue.

Nausea and other gastrointestinal symptoms are also common in breast cancer patients undergoing treatment. Palliative care providers may prescribe medications to help manage these symptoms, as well as recommend dietary changes or other lifestyle modifications to help alleviate nausea.

Palliative care plays an essential role in managing the physical, emotional, and psychosocial symptoms that can arise in patients with prostate cancer. Some of the most common challenges facing patients with prostate cancer include pain, fatigue, sexual dysfunction, and emotional distress.

Example: Palliative care for prostate cancer patients

One solution for managing pain in patients with prostate cancer is medication management. Depending on the severity of the pain and the patient's medical history, doctors may prescribe opioids or other pain medications to manage pain. Other pain management strategies may include nerve blocks, physical therapy, or other non-pharmacological interventions.

Fatigue is another common symptom experienced by patients with prostate cancer. Palliative care providers may recommend lifestyle modifications, such as exercise or rest, to help manage fatigue. Addressing underlying factors such as anemia or sleep disorders may also help to reduce fatigue.

Sexual dysfunction is also a common symptom experienced by patients with prostate cancer. Palliative care providers can help manage sexual dysfunction by offering counseling, providing information about sexual aids or devices, or recommending medications that may improve sexual function.

Emotional distress is another significant challenge faced by patients with prostate cancer. Palliative care providers may offer counseling or other psychosocial interventions to help patients manage emotional distress, anxiety, and depression. Family members may also benefit from counseling or support services to help them cope with the emotional impact of prostate cancer.

The outcome of effective palliative care for patients with any cancer can be improved quality of life, reduced symptoms, and improved psychological well-being for both the patient and their family. Patients may be able to continue with their daily activities, such as work or hobbies, with less interference from symptoms. Family members may also feel more supported and less overwhelmed by the caregiving responsibilities. Overall, palliative care can help to improve the patient's experience of living with cancer, regardless of the stage of the disease.

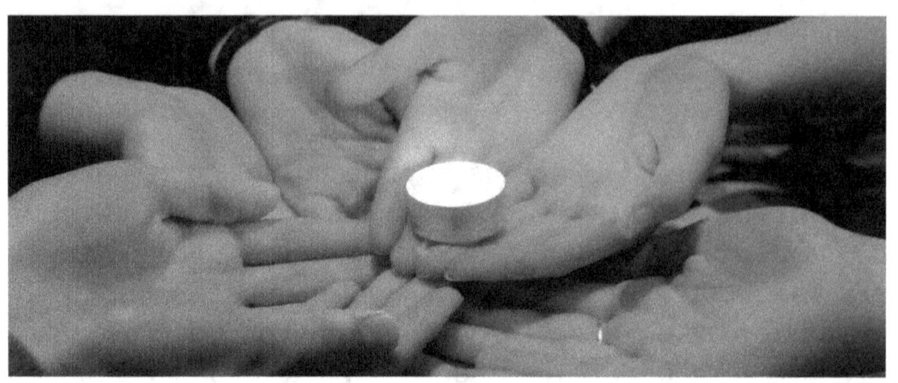

CHAPTER 20 CATERING PALLIATIVE CARE TO A SPECIFIC CANCER TREATMENT PROVIDED

Palliative care should not be a one-size-fits-all approach for cancer patients because the disease itself and its treatments can vary greatly from person to person. Different types and stages of cancer present distinct challenges and symptoms, requiring tailored interventions. Additionally, individual responses to treatment, pain levels, emotional needs, and personal preferences can differ significantly. By recognizing the unique aspects of each patient's cancer diagnosis and providing personalized palliative care, healthcare providers can address specific symptoms, manage treatment side effects, alleviate pain, and offer appropriate psychosocial support, ultimately enhancing the quality of life for cancer patients and their families.

Palliative care for cancer patients undergoing surgery

Palliative care can be provided to cancer patients who are undergoing surgery in a number of ways. Here are a few examples:

1. Pain management: One of the main goals of palliative care is to manage symptoms, including pain. This can be especially important for cancer patients who may experience pain before and after surgery. Palliative care providers can work with the patient's surgeon and medical team to develop a pain management plan that takes into account the patient's individual needs and preferences.

2. Emotional support: Surgery can be stressful and emotionally challenging for cancer patients. Palliative care providers can offer emotional support to patients and their families, providing counseling or connecting them with support groups or other resources.

3. Education: Palliative care providers can provide education to cancer patients undergoing surgery about what to expect before, during, and after the procedure. This can include information about potential side effects or complications, as well as tips for managing recovery at home.

4. Advance care planning: Palliative care providers can help cancer patients undergoing surgery with advance care planning, which involves discussing the patient's goals and preferences for end-of-life care. This can help ensure that the patient's wishes are respected in the event of a medical emergency or deterioration in health.

5. Spiritual and cultural support: Palliative care providers can offer spiritual or cultural support to patients who may have specific needs related to their beliefs or cultural background.

Overall, the goal of palliative care for cancer patients undergoing surgery is to provide support, manage symptoms, and improve the patient's overall quality of life. By taking a holistic approach that considers the patient's physical, emotional, and spiritual needs, palliative care providers can help cancer patients navigate this challenging time with greater comfort and peace of mind.

here's a table outlining some potential medications used in

palliative care for cancer patients receiving surgery, along with their potential benefits:

Medication	Potential Benefits
Opioids (e.g. morphine, fentanyl)	Effective pain relief
Nonsteroidal anti-inflammatory drugs (NSAIDs)	Reduces inflammation and provides pain relief
Antidepressants (e.g. tricyclic antidepressants, selective serotonin reuptake inhibitors)	Helps manage depression, anxiety, and neuropathic pain
Anticonvulsants (e.g. gabapentin, pregabalin)	Helps manage neuropathic pain and prevent seizures
Steroids (e.g. dexamethasone)	Reduces inflammation and swelling
Bisphosphonates (e.g. zoledronic acid)	Helps prevent bone loss and fractures
Antiemetics (e.g. ondansetron)	Helps manage nausea and vomiting

Palliative care for cancer patients receiving radiation therapy

Radiation therapy is a common treatment for cancer that can cause various physical and emotional side effects. Palliative care can be beneficial for cancer patients going through radiation therapy, as it aims to improve their overall quality of life and manage their symptoms. Here are some ways to provide palliative care to cancer patients going through radiation therapy:

1. Pain management: Radiation therapy can cause pain, discomfort, and skin irritation. Pain medications and topical

creams can help manage these symptoms and improve the patient's comfort.

2. Nutritional support: Radiation therapy can affect the patient's appetite and ability to eat. A nutritionist can provide advice and support to help the patient maintain a healthy diet and manage side effects such as nausea and vomiting.

3. Emotional support: Radiation therapy can be stressful and emotionally challenging. A social worker, therapist, or support group can provide emotional support and help the patient cope with the anxiety and uncertainty associated with treatment.

4. Skin care: Radiation therapy can cause skin irritation and dryness. Moisturizers and ointments can help soothe the skin and prevent further damage.

5. Education: Education is an essential part of palliative care for cancer patients going through radiation therapy. Patients should receive information about the treatment process, potential side effects, and strategies for managing symptoms.

6. Spiritual and cultural support: Patients may have spiritual or cultural needs that should be addressed during radiation therapy. Spiritual care providers can help patients and their families cope with the emotional and spiritual aspects of the disease.

It's important to note that these are just a few examples of palliative care options for cancer patients going through radiation therapy. Palliative care is always tailored to the individual needs of the patient and may involve a wide range of services and interventions. The goal is to provide comprehensive support to patients and their families throughout the entire radiation therapy process.

Here is a table outlining some potential medications used in palliative care for cancer patients receiving radiation therapy, along with their potential benefits:

Medication	Potential Benefits
Opioids	Relief from pain and discomfort
Antiemetics	Prevention or relief of nausea and vomiting
Topical analgesics	Relief from skin irritation and discomfort
Antidepressants	Improvement of mood and management of anxiety or depression
Benzodiazepines	Reduction of anxiety and promotion of relaxation
Steroids	Reduction of inflammation and swelling
Bisphosphonates	Prevention or treatment of bone pain and bone loss
Laxatives	Management of constipation
Antihistamines	Relief of itching and allergic reactions
Antipsychotics	Management of delirium or agitation
Sleep aids	Promotion of restful sleep
Stool softeners	Management of constipation and prevention of straining during bowel movements

Palliative care for cancer patients receiving chemotherapy

Palliative care for cancer patients going through chemotherapy aims to manage the physical and emotional symptoms that arise as a result of the treatment. Below are some ways in which palliative care can be provided to patients undergoing chemotherapy:

1. Pain management: Chemotherapy can cause pain and discomfort, so pain management is a critical component of palliative care for cancer patients. Pain medication can range from over-the-counter medications such as acetaminophen and NSAIDs, to prescription opioids.

2. Nutritional support: Chemotherapy can often lead to loss of appetite, nausea, vomiting, and weight loss. Nutritional support in the form of dietary counseling, appetite stimulants, and anti-nausea medications can help alleviate these symptoms.

3. Emotional support: Cancer patients undergoing chemotherapy often experience a range of emotional symptoms such as anxiety, depression, and fear. Counseling, support groups, and medications such as antidepressants can help manage these symptoms.

4. Symptom management: Chemotherapy can cause a variety of symptoms such as fatigue, neuropathy, and skin reactions. Palliative care interventions such as physical therapy, topical creams, and ointments can help manage these symptoms.

5. Education: Providing information about the chemotherapy treatment process, potential side effects, and symptom management can help patients feel more informed and empowered during their treatment.

6. Spiritual and cultural support: Addressing the spiritual and cultural needs of cancer patients undergoing chemotherapy is an important aspect of palliative care. Spiritual care providers and cultural advisors can provide support and guidance in this area.

A comprehensive approach to palliative care for cancer patients undergoing chemotherapy involves tailoring interventions to the specific needs of the individual patient. Palliative care providers work closely with the patient's oncology team to ensure that their symptoms and needs are being addressed effectively.

Here is a table outlining some potential medications used in palliative care for cancer patients receiving chemotherapy, along with their potential benefits

Medication	Potential Benefits
Acetaminophen	Relieves pain and reduces fever
Nonsteroidal anti-inflammatory drugs (NSAIDs)	Relieves pain, reduces inflammation, and lowers fever
Opioids (e.g. morphine, fentanyl)	Relieves moderate to severe pain
Anti-nausea medications (e.g. ondansetron, metoclopramide)	Prevents or reduces nausea and vomiting
Steroids (e.g. dexamethasone)	Reduces inflammation, relieves pain, and improves appetite
Antidepressants (e.g. selective serotonin reuptake inhibitors)	Treats depression and anxiety
Anxiolytics (e.g. lorazepam)	Relieves anxiety and promotes sleep
Bisphosphonates (e.g. zoledronic acid)	Helps prevent bone loss and fractures
Erythropoiesis-stimulating agents (e.g. epoetin alfa)	Stimulates red blood cell production and reduces fatigue
Filgrastim	Stimulates white blood

> cell production and reduces the risk of infection

Palliative care for cancer patients undergoing targeted therapy

Palliative care for cancer patients undergoing targeted therapy involves addressing their physical, emotional, and social needs. Targeted therapy is a type of cancer treatment that uses drugs to specifically target cancer cells while minimizing damage to healthy cells. Common side effects of targeted therapy include fatigue, nausea, vomiting, skin rash, diarrhea, and loss of appetite. To provide palliative care for cancer patients undergoing targeted therapy, healthcare providers may:

1. Address physical symptoms: Healthcare providers may prescribe medications to manage symptoms such as nausea, vomiting, and diarrhea. They may also recommend dietary changes to improve appetite and prevent weight loss, and suggest exercises or physical therapy to improve strength and reduce fatigue.

2. Address emotional and psychological needs: Patients undergoing targeted therapy may experience anxiety, depression, and other emotional or psychological distress. Healthcare providers may offer counseling, support groups, or other resources to help patients cope with these feelings.

3. Provide social support: Cancer patients undergoing targeted therapy may face social isolation or financial stress due to their illness. Healthcare providers may connect patients with support groups or financial assistance programs to help alleviate these stressors.

4. Monitor for side effects: Healthcare providers will monitor patients for any potential side effects of targeted therapy and adjust treatment as needed. They may also provide education on

how to manage side effects at home.

5. Evaluate and adjust treatment goals: As with any palliative care, it is important to evaluate and adjust treatment goals based on the patient's preferences and needs. Palliative care should be individualized and patient centered.

In summary, providing palliative care to cancer patients undergoing targeted therapy involves addressing physical, emotional, and social needs, monitoring for side effects, and individualizing treatment goals based on the patient's preferences and needs.

Here is a table outlining some potential medications used in palliative care for cancer patients receiving targeted therapy, along with their potential benefits:

Medication	Potential Benefits
Anti-nausea medications (e.g., ondansetron, aprepitant)	Reduces nausea and vomiting
Skin moisturizers (e.g., emollients, urea cream)	Prevents or relieves skin rash and dryness
Steroids (e.g., dexamethasone)	Reduces inflammation and swelling
Antidepressants (e.g., sertraline, duloxetine)	Improves mood and reduces anxiety and depression
Anti-anxiety medications (e.g., lorazepam, alprazolam)	Reduces anxiety and promotes relaxation
Nonsteroidal anti-inflammatory drugs (NSAIDs) (e.g., ibuprofen)	Reduces pain and inflammation
Opioids (e.g., morphine, fentanyl)	Reduces pain

Stimulants (e.g., methylphenidate, modafinil)	Reduces fatigue and improves alertness
Bisphosphonates (e.g., zoledronic acid)	Prevents or treats bone loss and fractures
Anticoagulants (e.g., enoxaparin)	Prevents blood clots

Palliative care for cancer patients receiving immunotherapy

Palliative care for cancer patients receiving immunotherapy involves managing symptoms and side effects related to the treatment. Some potential strategies for providing palliative care to cancer patients going through immunotherapy include:

1. Addressing side effects: Immunotherapy can cause a range of side effects, including fatigue, nausea, fever, rash, and diarrhea. Palliative care providers can work with the patient's oncologist to manage these symptoms and provide supportive care to improve the patient's overall quality of life.

2. Managing pain: Immunotherapy can also cause pain, particularly in patients with bone or liver metastases. Pain management strategies may include non-opioid pain medications, such as nonsteroidal anti-inflammatory drugs (NSAIDs) or acetaminophen, or opioid pain medications for more severe pain.

3. Providing emotional support: Cancer patients receiving immunotherapy may experience a range of emotional challenges, including anxiety, depression, and fear of treatment failure. Palliative care providers can offer emotional support and counseling to help patients cope with these feelings and maintain a positive outlook.

4. Nutritional support: Immunotherapy can cause loss of appetite, nausea, and vomiting, which can lead to malnutrition

and weight loss. Palliative care providers can work with the patient's oncologist and dietitian to provide nutritional support and ensure the patient is getting the nutrients they need to maintain their strength and energy.

5. Providing end-of-life care: In some cases, immunotherapy may not be effective in controlling the cancer, and patients may require end-of-life care. Palliative care providers can work with the patient and their family to provide comfort care and support during this time.

Overall, the goal of palliative care for cancer patients going through immunotherapy is to improve the patient's quality of life by addressing symptoms and side effects related to treatment and providing emotional support and counseling. The specific palliative care strategies used will depend on the individual patient's needs and treatment plan.

Here is a table outlining some potential medications used in palliative care for cancer patients receiving immunotherapy, along with their potential benefits:

Medication	Potential Benefits
Corticosteroids (e.g. prednisone)	Reduction of inflammation and swelling, improvement of appetite, relief of pain, reduction of fatigue and nausea
Antiemetics (e.g. ondansetron)	Reduction of nausea and vomiting
Immunomodulatory agents (e.g. thalidomide)	Reduction of inflammation and improvement of quality of life
Pain relievers (e.g. opioids)	Relief of pain and improvement of quality of

	life
Benzodiazepines (e.g. lorazepam)	Reduction of anxiety and improvement of sleep
Antidepressants (e.g. fluoxetine)	Reduction of depression and anxiety
Psychostimulants (e.g. methylphenidate)	Reduction of fatigue and improvement of cognitive function
Bisphosphonates (e.g. zoledronic acid)	Prevention and treatment of bone metastases and reduction of bone pain

Example of Palliative Care on Hair loss from Chemotherapy

Hair loss is a common side effect of chemotherapy treatment for breast cancer patients. This can be emotionally difficult for patients, as changes in appearance can affect self-esteem and quality of life. As a part of palliative care, there are several solutions available to address hair loss and help breast cancer patients cope with this side effect:

1. Scalp cooling: One solution that has been shown to be effective in reducing hair loss is scalp cooling. This involves using a cooling cap during chemotherapy treatment to reduce blood flow to the scalp, which can help protect hair follicles from damage.

2. Wigs and head coverings: Many breast cancer patients choose to wear wigs or other head coverings to cover hair loss. There are many options available, from synthetic wigs to real hair wigs, scarves, hats, and turbans.

3. Education and support: Healthcare providers can educate breast cancer patients on the side effects of chemotherapy,

including hair loss, and provide support and guidance on how to cope with these changes in appearance.

4. Cosmetic solutions: There are cosmetic solutions available, such as makeup and eyebrow pencils, that can help breast cancer patients enhance their appearance and feel more confident.

5. Emotional support: Emotional support is an important aspect of palliative care. Breast cancer patients may benefit from counseling or support groups to help cope with the emotional impact of hair loss and cancer treatment.

It is important for healthcare providers to address hair loss as a part of palliative care for breast cancer patients undergoing chemotherapy. By providing education, support, and solutions, healthcare providers can help breast cancer patients cope with hair loss and maintain their quality of life.

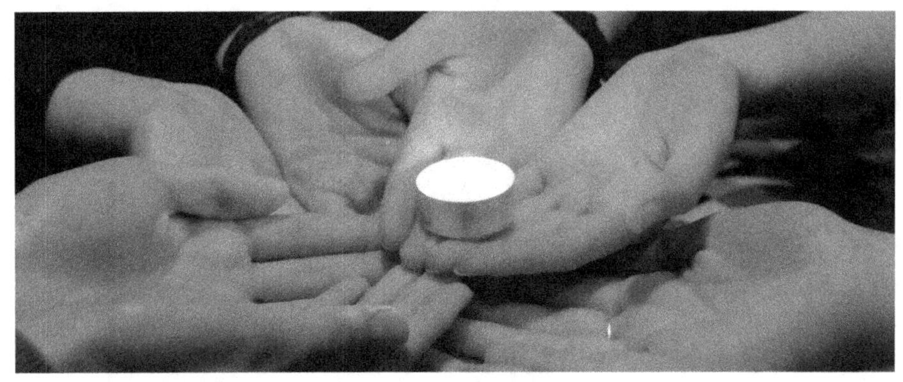

CHAPTER 21 HOSPICE CARE

Hospice care is a specialized type of medical care that is focused on providing comfort and support to patients who have been diagnosed with a terminal illness, such as cancer. Hospice care is designed to provide physical, emotional, and spiritual care through comfort, support and dignity to patients and their families in their final days, weeks, or months of life. Various aspects of hospice care for cancer patients include planning, family member considerations, personal wishes, dealing with physical and emotional pain, and after-death arrangements.

Planning for Hospice Care

When a patient is diagnosed with cancer and has been told that curative treatment options are no longer available, it is important to consider hospice care. Hospice care can be provided in a variety of settings, including in the patient's home, at a hospice facility, or in a hospital. The decision about where to receive hospice care will depend on the patient's needs and wishes, as well as the availability of resources.

Hospice care providers typically include a team of healthcare professionals, including physicians, nurses, social workers, and chaplains. They work together to provide physical, emotional, and spiritual support to the patient and their family. The hospice team will develop a personalized care plan for the patient, which will include medications to manage pain and other symptoms, as well as strategies to address emotional and spiritual needs.

Family Member Consideration

Hospice care is not just for the patient; it is also designed to support the patient's family members. Family members may be asked to participate in the patient's care, including administering medications, feeding, bathing and providing emotional support. The hospice team can also provide counseling and support to family members, helping them to take care of themselves as well as cope with the stress and grief associated with their loved one's illness and impending death.

Personal Wishes

One of the benefits of hospice care is that it allows patients to maintain control over their lives and make decisions about their care. Patients can express their personal wishes and preferences about their care, including what type of medical interventions they want and what kind of cultural, spiritual and emotional support they need. Hospice providers will work with the patient and their family to honor these wishes aligned with the patient's values and preferences and ensure that the patient's unique needs are met.

Dealing with Physical and Emotional Pain

Pain management is an important part of hospice care for cancer patients. Hospice providers use a variety of medications and other strategies to manage pain and other symptoms, such as nausea, vomiting, and shortness of breath. This may include medication, physical therapy, massage, or other complementary therapies.

In addition, hospice providers can offer emotional and spiritual support to patients and their families, helping them to cope with the anxiety, depression, and other emotional issues that arise during this difficult time.

After Death

Hospice care continues after the patient's death. After the patient has passed away, hospice providers can assist the family with making arrangements for funeral or memorial services. They can also provide bereavement counseling and support to help family members cope with their grief and loss.

In conclusion, hospice care is a critical component of end-of-life care for patients with cancer. Hospice care provides physical, emotional, and spiritual support to patients and their families during the final stages of life. It is important for patients and their families to begin planning for hospice care as soon as possible to ensure that the care provided is aligned with the patient's wishes and preferences. Hospice care providers work closely with patients and their families to provide care that is tailored to the patient's unique needs, and help patients and their families find peace and comfort during this final chapter of life.

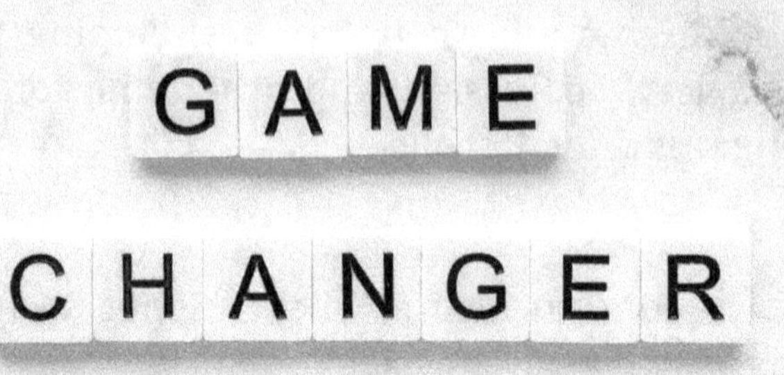

SECTION VII CREATING AN ACTION PLAN AFTER CANCER DIAGNOSIS

Benjamin Franklin once said: "If you fail to plan, you plan to fail." Fighting against cancer is like a war and needs careful planning. For a newly diagnosed cancer patient, the sooner an action plan is in place, the better his(her) chance of success (s)he has in defeating cancer. Below is a table outlining an action plan for a newly diagnosed cancer patient, which we are going into more detail in this section.

Action	Brief Description	Party Responsible
Seek Support	Seek emotional support from friends, family, or a professional therapist. Join a support group for people with cancer.	Patient, Friends/Family, Therapist
Understand the Diagnosis	Understand the type and stage of cancer, as well as the recommended treatment options. Ask healthcare provider questions and request additional information as	Patient, Healthcare Provider

	needed.	
Find a Treatment Team	Seek out a team of healthcare providers who specialize in cancer treatment, such as an oncologist, surgeon, and radiation oncologist. Consider getting a second opinion.	Patient, Healthcare Provider
Prepare for Treatment	Discuss potential side effects of treatment with healthcare provider and develop a plan to manage them. Prepare for any logistical considerations, such as time off from work or childcare arrangements.	Patient, Healthcare Provider
Consider a Backup Plan	Develop a backup plan in case the initial treatment plan does not work or if there are unexpected complications. This may include alternative treatment options, such as clinical trials, or a plan for palliative care.	Patient, Healthcare Provider
Take Care of Mental and Emotional Health	Prioritize self-care and stress-reducing activities, such as exercise, meditation, or spending time with loved ones. Maintain regular communication with the treatment team and seek help if feelings of depression or anxiety become overwhelming.	Patient, Therapist
Communicate with Loved Ones	Communicate openly with loved ones about the	Patient, Friends/ Family

> diagnosis, treatment plan,
> and any concerns or fears.
> Involve loved ones in the
> decision-making process
> and ask for their support
> throughout the treatment
> journey.

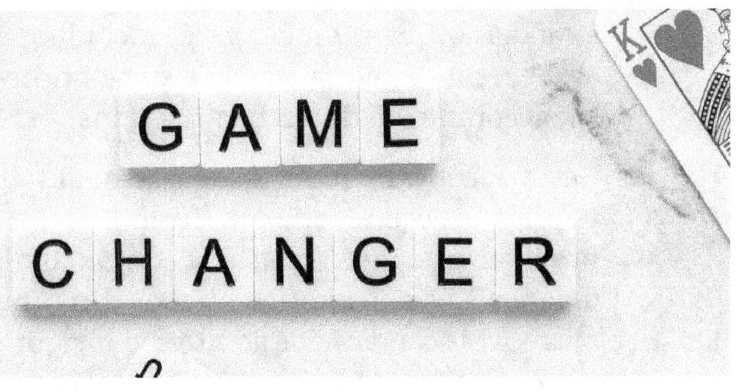

CHAPTER 22 UNDERSTAND THE DIAGNOSIS AND CHOOSE A TRUSTED TREATMENT TEAM

Understanding the type and stage of cancer can help a patient feel more in control of their diagnosis. When a patient has a clear understanding of their diagnosis, they may feel more empowered to take an active role in their treatment and make decisions that are right for them. Understanding the type and stage of cancer can also help a patient know what to expect during treatment and recovery. For example, they can learn about potential side effects of treatment, how long treatment may last, and what the likelihood of recovery is, in turn which can help a patient make informed decisions about their treatment options.

There are several steps a patient can take to understand the type and stage of cancer, including:

1. Ask the healthcare provider: Patients can ask their healthcare provider who made the initial diagnosis for more information about the type and stage of cancer. The healthcare provider should provide a detailed

explanation of the diagnosis, including the location and extent of the cancer, the stage of the cancer, and the recommended treatment options.

2. Get a second opinion: Patients should also consider getting a second opinion from another healthcare provider or cancer specialist, especially if the initial diagnosis was made at a rural or community medical office. This can provide additional insight and help the patient make a more informed decision about their treatment options.

3. Research online: Meeting with a healthcare provider needs advanced scheduling and the meeting time is usually limited, potentially leaving a patient with unanswered questions. Patients can do their own research online back at home to learn more about their specific type of cancer and its stage. There are many reliable websites and resources that provide detailed information about cancer, including the National Cancer Institute, American Cancer Society, Cancer.Net and Cancer Research UK.

4. Attend cancer support groups offline and/or online: Many cancer support groups offer educational sessions where patients can learn about their diagnosis and ask questions. Support groups can also provide emotional support and help patients connect with others who are going through a similar experience. A table of groups on Facebook supporting cancer patients is listed below. It is important to note that not all resources found online may be reliable, but patients can set up follow-up meetings with their healthcare provider for clarification and advice.

5. Talk to other cancer survivors: Patients should also talk to other cancer survivors who have had a similar type and stage of cancer. Ask your healthcare provider

to see if other cancer survivors are willing to share their experiences. This can provide valuable insight into what to expect during treatment and recovery and offer emotional support.

Researching Online

To research online, a cancer patient can use the websites listed below to find reliable information on cancer, cancer staging and related topics.

Website	Description
American Cancer Society (https://www.cancer.org/)	Provides information on a wide range of cancer topics, including cancer types, treatments, coping with cancer, and support for patients and caregivers. Also includes detailed information on cancer staging and prognosis.
National Cancer Institute (https://www.cancer.gov/)	Provides up-to-date information on cancer research, clinical

	trials, cancer statistics, and cancer treatment options. Also includes resources for patients and caregivers on coping with cancer and managing side effects.
Cancer.Net (https://www.cancer.net/)	Provides patient-friendly information on cancer types, treatment options, and coping with cancer. Also includes information on clinical trials, cancer staging, and survivorship.
Mayo Clinic (https://www.mayoclinic.org/)	Provides in-depth information on cancer types, symptoms, diagnosis, and

	treatment options. Also includes information on managing side effects, nutritional support, and complementary therapies.
Memorial Sloan Kettering Cancer Center (https://www.mskcc.org/)	Provides comprehensive information on cancer types, diagnosis, treatment options, and support for patients and caregivers. Also includes information on cancer staging, prognosis, and survivorship.
Oncology Nursing Society (https://www.ons.org/)	Provides resources for patients and caregivers on managing cancer treatment, including side effects,

	nutrition, and emotional support. Also includes information on cancer types and treatment options.
Cancer Research UK (https://www.cancerresearchuk.org/)	Provides information on cancer types, treatments, and research. Also includes resources for patients and caregivers on coping with cancer, managing side effects, and finding support.
Cancer Council Australia (https://www.cancer.org.au/)	Provides information on cancer types, prevention, diagnosis, and treatment options. Also includes resources for patients and caregivers

<table>
<tr><td></td><td>on coping with cancer, managing side effects, and finding support.</td></tr>
</table>

For example, the American Society of Clinical Oncology (ASCO) is the world's leading professional organization for physicians and oncology professionals caring for people with cancer. It has a dedicated webpage specifically for cancer patients and survivors at www.cancer.net where it offers individualized guides for more than 120 types of cancer and related hereditary syndromes. Each guide provides comprehensive, oncologist-approved information on: Introduction, Medical Illustrations, Risk Factors, Prevention, Symptoms & Signs, Diagnosis, Stages, Types of Treatment, About Clinical Trials, Latest Research, Coping with Treatment, Follow-Up Care, Survivorship, Questions to Ask the Health Care Team, and Additional Resources.

Joining a Cancer Support Groups

There are many cancer support groups that can be extremely helpful for a cancer patient going through the diagnosis and treatment. Here is a table listing some prominent cancer support groups.

Group Name	Description
Cancer Support Community	A large online community for cancer patients, survivors, and caregivers. Members can share their stories, ask questions, and offer support to one another.

Cancer Survivors Network	A group run by the American Cancer Society that provides a platform for cancer survivors to connect with one another. Members can share their stories, ask for advice, and offer support to others going through a similar experience.
Breast Cancer Support Group	A group specifically for women with breast cancer. Members can share their experiences, ask for advice, and connect with others going through a similar experience.
Lung Cancer Support Group	A group for individuals with lung cancer and their caregivers. Members can share their experiences, ask questions, and offer support to one another.
Gynecologic Cancer Support Group	A group for individuals with gynecologic cancers such as ovarian, cervical, and uterine cancer. Members can share their stories, ask for advice, and connect with others who have had a similar diagnosis.
Prostate Cancer Support Group	A group for individuals with prostate cancer and their caregivers. Members can share their experiences, ask questions, and offer support to one another.
Childhood Cancer	A group for parents and

Support Group	caregivers of children with cancer. Members can share their experiences, ask for advice, and connect with others who are going through a similar experience.
Brain Tumor Support Group	A group for individuals with brain tumors and their caregivers. Members can share their experiences, ask questions, and offer support to one another.
Colorectal Cancer Support Group	A group for individuals with colorectal cancer and their caregivers. Members can share their experiences, ask for advice, and connect with others who have had a similar diagnosis.
Pancreatic Cancer Support Group	A group for individuals with pancreatic cancer and their caregivers. Members can share their experiences, ask questions, and offer support to one another.
Multiple Myeloma Support Group	A group for individuals with multiple myeloma and their caregivers. Members can share their experiences, ask questions, and offer support to one another.
Bladder Cancer Support Group	A group for individuals with bladder cancer and their caregivers. Members can share their experiences, ask questions, and offer support to one another.

Sarcoma Support Group	A group for individuals with sarcoma and their caregivers. Members can share their experiences, ask questions, and offer support to one another.
Blood Cancer Support Group	A group for individuals with blood cancers such as leukemia, lymphoma, and myeloma. Members can share their experiences, ask for advice, and connect with others going through a similar experience.

Selecting a Trusted and Highly Experienced Cancer Treatment Team

While the cancer patient is spending time to understand more about the cancer type and stage, it is critical for the patient to select a trusted and highly experienced treatment team that can provide the best possible care and support throughout the treatment journey. The benefits of a trusted and highly experienced treatment team include:

1. Accurate Diagnosis: A highly experienced treatment team can ensure that the cancer diagnosis is accurate and complete. An accurate diagnosis is essential for determining the most appropriate treatment options and ensuring that the treatment is effective.

2. Personalized Treatment: A highly experienced treatment team will develop a personalized treatment plan that takes into account the patient's unique needs, preferences, and medical history. This can lead to better treatment outcomes and a higher quality of life for the patient.

3. Coordination of Care: A highly experienced treatment team can coordinate all aspects of the patient's care, including surgery, chemotherapy, radiation therapy, targeted therapy and immunotherapy. This can help to minimize the risk of complications and ensure that the patient receives the right treatment at the right time.

4. Emotional Support: Cancer treatment can be emotionally challenging, and a trusted treatment team can provide patients with emotional support and counseling. This will help patients cope with the stress and anxiety of cancer treatment and improve their overall quality of life.

5. Access to Clinical Trials: A highly experienced treatment team can provide patients with access to clinical trials and new treatment options that may not be available elsewhere. This can help patients receive cutting-edge treatments and potentially improve their outcomes.

An oncologist is the lead doctor on the treatment team, and depending on the cancer stage and treatment selection, the oncologist could be a cancer surgeon, a radiation oncologist and/or a medical oncologist. The experience of this oncologist will play probably the biggest role in deciding the treatment outcome. The table below lists the three most important questions regarding an oncologist's experience, and the patient can expand more on questions to ask if and when the oncologist is board certified, the availability of the doctor, and the range of treatment options available for your cancer, including standard treatments and any new or experimental treatments. The patient should also ask the doctor about the support services available to you and your family from the treatment facility, such as counseling, support groups, and financial assistance.

Type of Oncologist	Tips	Questions to Ask	Red Flags
Medical Oncologist	Ask for referrals, research online, check for board certification	How many patients with my type of cancer have you treated? What is your experience treating my type of cancer? What are your success rates?	Lack of board certification, lack of experience, poor communication
Cancer Surgeon	Ask for referrals, research online, check for board certification	How many surgeries have you performed for my type of cancer? What is your experience performing my type of surgery? What are your success rates?	Lack of board certification, lack of experience, poor communication
Radiation Oncologist	Ask for referrals, research online, check for board certification	How many patients with my type of cancer have you treated with radiation therapy? What is your experience treating my type of cancer with radiation therapy? What are your success rates?	Lack of board certification, lack of experience, poor communication

It is usually a good idea to have a second opinion after initial cancer diagnosis, and the cancer patient should use this opportunity as part of the process to select a trusted and highly experienced oncologist. Now for the cancer patient to come up with the initial 2-5 oncologist candidates for consideration, the patient can ask his(her) primary care physician or other healthcare professionals for recommendations. A slightly better option is to ask friends or family members who have gone through cancer treatment for their recommendations. The patient can also use online resources like the American Cancer Society's website or the National Cancer Institute's website to find comprehensive cancer centers in/near your area. As mentioned in Chapter 16, at NCI website https://www.cancer.gov/research/infrastructure/cancer-centers/find one can find 71 NCI-designated cancer centers that deliver cutting-edge cancer treatments to patients in communities across the United States. From there, one can check the doctors in one's insurance plan and start checking their credentials, experience, and areas of expertise. Alternatively, the cancer patients can go straight to the top 20 cancer centers ranked on cancer type by US News & World Report, which are listed in Chapter 16, and start researching oncologists from there.

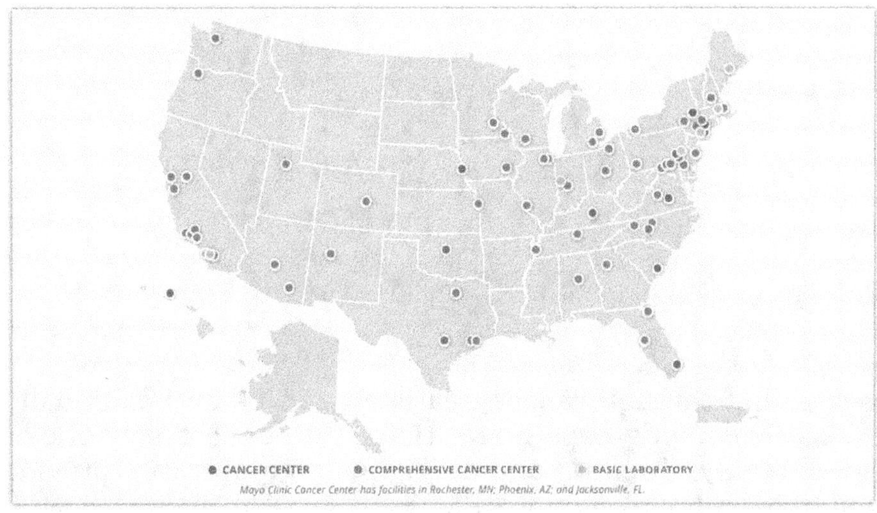

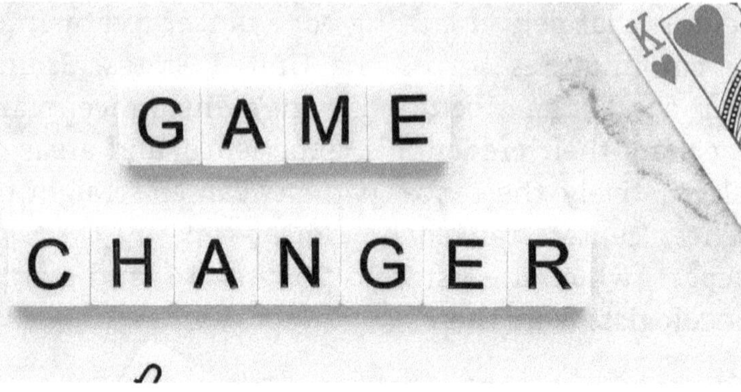

CHAPTER 23 BUILD A SOLID SUPPORT NETWORK AND PREPARE FOR TREATMENT

Going through cancer treatment can be an emotionally challenging experience. Having a support network of family, friends, and/or support groups can provide emotional support, comfort, and encouragement to help the patient cope with the emotional ups and downs of cancer treatment. In turn these will help the patient feel less isolated and more connected to others, help reduce stress levels for the patient, and have a positive impact on their overall health and well-being. Studies have shown that cancer patients who have strong social support systems are less likely to experience depression and anxiety.

Additionally, a support network can also provide practical support, such as helping with household chores, cooking meals, and providing transportation to appointments. For example, American Cancer Society has a patient program called "Road to Recovery" in several communities providing transportation to and from treatment for people with cancer who do not have a ride or are unable to drive themselves; American Cancer Society also has a "Patient Lodging Program" with 30+ Hope Lodge locations throughout the US and Puerto Rico providing free lodging for cancer patients and their caregivers when cancer treatment is far away from home, serving about 29,000 cancer patients and caregivers each year. Finally, A support network can provide the patient with reassuring information and advice about their treatment options, side effects, and how to manage symptoms. This can help the patient make informed decisions about their treatment and feel more in control of their situation. Here's a table with tips on how to build a support network for a cancer patient:

Action	Tips
Reach out to family and friends	Let them know about the diagnosis and how they can help. Ask them to come over, help with tasks, and simply spend time with you.
Join a support group	Find a support group for cancer patients or caregivers in your area. You can also join online communities or forums.
Talk to a social worker or patient navigator	They can connect you with local resources and support, including counseling services, financial assistance, and support groups.
Consider online support	Look for cancer-specific websites or social media groups to connect with others who are going through a similar experience.

Ask healthcare providers for recommendations	Your healthcare team can recommend local resources and support, such as support groups or counseling services.
Consider professional counseling	Counseling can provide additional emotional support and help patients and caregivers cope with the challenges of cancer treatment.

Some great examples of cancer-specific websites or social media groups are listed in the table below:

Resource	Description	Website Address
American Cancer Society	A nonprofit organization that provides information and resources about cancer, including treatment options, support groups, and education programs. They have an active social media presence on Facebook, Twitter, and Instagram.	https://www.cancer.org/
CancerCare	A nonprofit organization that provides free professional support services to people affected by cancer, including online support groups, counseling, and education programs. Their website has a searchable database of support groups and other resources.	https://www.cancercare.org/
Cancer Support Community	A nonprofit organization that provides free support services to cancer	https://www.cancersupportcommunity.org/

	patients and their families, including online support groups, counseling, and education programs. Their website has a searchable database of support groups and events, as well as other resources.	
Livestrong	A nonprofit organization that provides support and resources to people affected by cancer, including information about cancer, treatment options, and survivorship. They have an active social media presence on Facebook, Twitter, and Instagram.	https://www.livestrong.org/
CancerConnect	An online community for cancer patients and their families, with discussion forums, news, and information about treatment options and research.	https://news.cancerconnect.com/
Cancer Survivors Network	An online community for cancer survivors, with discussion forums, blogs, and resources for survivors and their families.	https://csn.cancer.org/
Cancer Support Community's MyLifeLine	An online platform that allows cancer patients and caregivers to create a free personalized website to share updates, coordinate care, and connect with others.	https://www.mylifeline.org/

Each of these organizations have their own strengths, and it is a good idea to check out all these websites to select the services a cancer patient might need. An infographic of CancerCare's impact is shown below.

CancerCare Impact for Fiscal Year 2022

Our oncology social workers answered **38,841 calls** to our helplines.

CancerCare provided

171,885

services to people affected by cancer.

CancerCare staff provided **31,569 hours of emotional and practical support**.

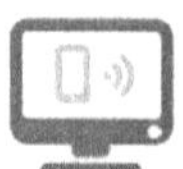

144 experts led **80 CancerCare Connect® Education Workshops**, drawing **44,043 participants** with the help of **97 partner organizations**.

957,511

Distributed publications to people living with cancer, caregivers, loved ones and professionals.

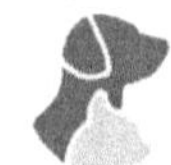

The Pet Assistance & Wellness (PAW) Program helped **463 clients** keep their pet in the home.

CancerCare provided **$81 million** in financial and co-payment assistance to **28,664 people** for costs including transportation and practical needs and to help pay for cancer medications.

CancerCare welcomed

1.8 million

visits to our websites.

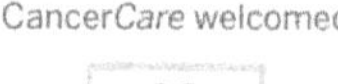

CANCERcare
Over 25 Years of Help and Hope

Providing free, professional support for anyone affected by cancer.

800-813-HOPE (4673) | WWW.CANCERCARE.ORG

July 1, 2021 – June 30, 2022

Besides building a strong support network, cancer patients also need to take care of their mental and emotional health. Here are some additional tips for taking care of mental and emotional health for a cancer patient:

1. Seek support: Reach out to family, friends, and support groups you are building to talk about your feelings and concerns. Connecting with people who understand what you're going through can help you feel less isolated and provides a sense of comfort and support.

2. Practice self-care: It's important to take care of yourself physically and emotionally during this time. This can include getting enough rest, eating a healthy diet, engaging in regular exercise, and participating in activities that bring you joy.

3. Talk to a mental health professional: Consider seeing

a mental health professional, such as a counselor or therapist, who can help you cope with the emotional challenges of cancer. They can provide you with tools and strategies for managing stress, anxiety, depression, and other emotional issues.

4. Engage in relaxation techniques: Relaxation techniques, such as deep breathing, meditation, or yoga, can help reduce stress and anxiety and promote feelings of calmness and relaxation. Work with healthcare providers to enhance engagement.

5. Stay informed, but don't obsess: It's important to stay informed about your cancer and treatment, but obsessively researching or focusing on the disease can be overwhelming. Find a balance that works for you and take breaks when needed.

6. Allow yourself to feel and express your emotions: It's okay to feel a range of emotions, including sadness, anger, and fear. Allow yourself to feel and express these emotions in healthy ways, such as through talking, writing, or creative outlets.

While asking for details on treatment options is a crucial part of the process for a cancer patient to select a treatment team, there are additional questions and activities that the patient must prepare for once the treatment starts.

According to NCI, a cancer patient may have many questions to ask during the treatment, such as:

- Where will I go for treatment?

- How is the treatment given?

- How long will each treatment session take?

- How many treatment sessions will I have?

- Should a family member or friend come with me to my treatment sessions?

- How will I feel after each treatment? Will I be able to go about my day or should I plan to rest?

- Will I be able to work? Should I think about going part-time?

- Will treatment affect my appetite or make it hard to eat?

- What are the possible side effects of the treatment?

- What side effects may happen during or between my treatment sessions?

- Are there any side effects that I should call you about right away?

- Are there any lasting side effects of the treatment?

- Will this treatment affect my ability to have children?

- Will treatment affect my appetite or make it hard to eat?

- How can I prevent or treat side effects?

- What should I do with my dietary supplement and nutritional plans?

- Could any drugs or supplements change the way that cancer treatment works?

Meanwhile, it is equally important for a cancer patient to know about the things to avoid during treatment.

What to avoid	Why to avoid

Delaying treatment	Cancer may spread and become more difficult to treat.
Skipping appointments	Appointments are crucial for monitoring progress and making any necessary adjustments to the treatment plan.
Ignoring side effects	Side effects may interfere with treatment and make the treatment process more challenging.
Not asking questions	Understanding the treatment plan and feeling empowered to make decisions can help the patient feel more in control.
Isolating oneself	Maintaining social connections and seeking

	support can help the patient cope with the emotional challenges of treatment.
Neglecting self-care like getting enough rest, eating a healthy diet, and engaging in regular exercise.	Taking care of oneself during treatment is crucial for physical and emotional well-being.
Using alternative therapies without consulting the healthcare team	Some alternative therapies may interfere with conventional cancer treatments.

Throughout the treatment process, a cancer patient needs to maintain a strong will to overcome potential side effects or setbacks. Cancer survivors who have beaten cancer have a lot of inspirational messages that are of hope, perseverance, and the power of the human spirit to overcome even the most challenging of obstacles. Here are some examples of inspirational sentences, phrases, and stories that cancer survivors have shared with others going through cancer treatment:

- "Believe in yourself and your ability to overcome this challenge."

- "You are not alone. We are here for you, and we will

support you through this journey."

- "One day at a time. Each day, you are one step closer to being cancer-free."

- "You are stronger than you know. You have already come so far, and you will continue to fight."

- "There is hope, even in the darkest of times. Keep fighting, keep pushing, and never give up."

- "Cancer does not define you. You are more than your diagnosis, and you will come out of this even stronger."

- "Celebrate every small victory along the way. Each milestone is a step closer to healing and recovery."

- "Take care of yourself, both physically and emotionally. It's okay to ask for help, and to take things one day at a time."

- "Remember that there is life after cancer. You will get through this, and you will come out the other side with a renewed sense of gratitude and purpose."

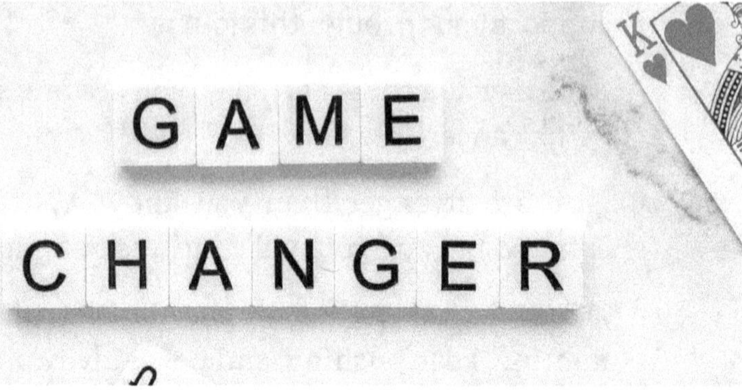

CHAPTER 24 CREATE A BACKUP PLAN AND COMMUNICATE WITH LOVED ONES

Having a backup plan for a cancer patient is important because not all treatments work for everyone. Cancer is a complex disease, and there are many factors that can affect how well a particular treatment works for an individual patient. Additionally, cancer can sometimes mutate or evolve in a way that makes it resistant to certain treatments.

If the initial treatment plan does not work, having a backup plan in place can help the patient and their healthcare team quickly pivot to an alternative approach. This can help avoid delays in treatment, which are especially important when it comes to cancer. Delays can give the cancer more time to grow and spread, which can make it more difficult to treat.

Having a backup plan can also help reduce anxiety and uncertainty for the patient and their loved ones. Cancer treatment can be an emotional rollercoaster, and the uncertainty of whether a treatment will work or not can be particularly challenging. Knowing that there is a backup plan in place can provide a sense of security and comfort.

The steps to develop a backup plan for a cancer patient are shown in the table below. Some related websites are also provided.

Step	Description	Related Websites
1. Talk to your healthcare team	Have an open and honest conversation with your healthcare team about the possibility of a backup plan. They can provide guidance on what options may be available and help you understand the potential risks and benefits of each.	American Cancer Society (https://www.cancer.org/) CancerCare (https://www.cancercare.org/)
2. Consider alternative treatments	If the initial treatment plan does not work, there may be alternative treatments that could be effective. For example, if chemotherapy is not working, radiation therapy or immunotherapy may be considered. Your healthcare team can help you understand the options that may be available.	National Cancer Institute (https://www.cancer.gov/) Cancer Research Institute (https://www.cancerresearch.org/)
3. Explore clinical trials	Clinical trials are studies that test new treatments for cancer. If the initial treatment plan is not effective, there may be a clinical trial that could offer a new approach. Your healthcare team can help you understand the clinical trial options that may be available and whether you may be eligible to participate.	ClinicalTrials.gov (https://clinicaltrials.gov/) National Cancer Institute (https://www.cancer.gov/)
4. Discuss palliative care	If the cancer is advanced or the treatments are no longer effective, it may be appropriate to	National Hospice and Palliative Care Organization (https://www.nhpco.org/) Hospice Foundation of America (https://hospicefoundation.org/)

	discuss palliative care options. Palliative care focuses on managing symptoms and improving quality of life, and may include pain management, nutrition support, and other types of supportive care.	
5. Consider second opinions	If you are unsure about the treatment plan or the backup plan, it may be helpful to seek a second opinion from another healthcare provider. They can provide a fresh perspective and help ensure that all options have been considered.	Cancer.net (https://www.cancer.net/) SecondOpinions.com (https://secondopinions.com/)

For example, Cancer Research Institute is a leader in immunotherapy, and the institute has hosted annual Immunotherapy Patient Summits which are free online virtual events that connect cancer patients and caregivers with scientific and medical experts to learn about emerging breakthroughs in cancer immunotherapy and clinical trials, with Interactive cancer-specific breakout sessions with leading experts, including breast cancer, lung cancer, prostate cancer, melanoma and bladder cancer. The virtual summit includes an overview of cancer immunotherapy clinical trials and how to access them, as well as virtual, confidential, one-on-one clinical trial navigator appointments.

Separately, Cancer.Net website, in its Research and Advocacy Section, has comprehensive information and lists regarding clinical trials that might be easier to research than ClinicalTrials.gov website. The clinical trial listings on Cancer.Net website have 3 parts worth checking out:

1. US Government clinical trials managed by ClinicalTrials.gov and NCI;

2. general clinical trial listings including EmergingMed clinical trial navigator service, Lazarex Cancer Foundation, CenterWatch and WHO International clinical trials registry;

3. Disease-specific clinical trial listings including BreastCancerTrials.org, Metastatic Breast Cancer Project, Metastatic Prostate Cancer Project, National Brain Tumor Society Clinical Trial Finder, Bladder Cancer Advocacy Network etc.

For a serious disease such as cancer, unfortunately there could be a time when the treatments are causing substantial side effects or are no longer effective, and the cancer patient will have to consider palliative care or hospice care options. The decision of which type of care to pursue ultimately depends on the patient's goals and wishes, as well as their overall health status and prognosis. It is important for patients and their families to have open and honest conversations with their healthcare team regarding the options when working on the backup plan. While both palliative care and hospice care can reduce patient suffering including pain and other physical symptoms, emotional and spiritual distress, stress and anxiety, as well as caregiver burden, there are some key differences between the two types of care, as shown in the table below. One thing to note is that the cancer patient can leave hospice care if a patient's condition improves, or they decide they wish to resume curative care and return to hospice care later.

	Palliative Care	**Hospice Care**
Focus	Improve quality of life by managing symptoms and stress	Provide comfort care for terminally ill patients
Medical treatment	Concurrent	Cease curative

	with curative treatments	treatments and focus on comfort care
Timing	Available at any stage of illness	Available when life expectancy is six months or less
Goal	To relieve symptoms and improve quality of life	To provide comfort and dignity for the patient and family
Location	Can be provided in any healthcare setting, hospital, outpatient clinic, or at home	Can be provided at home, hospice center, or hospital
Team	Multidisciplinary team including doctors and specialists	Team includes doctors, nurses, social workers, chaplains
Services	Pain and symptom management, emotional support	Pain and symptom management, emotional and spiritual support
Cost	Usually covered by insurance	Covered by Medicare,

		Medicaid, or private insurance
Decision-making	Patient can continue to make decisions about their care	Patient can still make decisions, but family may also help
Bereavement support	Available for family and loved ones	Available for family and loved ones after patient passes

Caringinfo (https://www.caringinfo.org), a program of the National Hospice and Palliative Care Organization, offers a large selection of guides and resources on specific topics like advance directive, palliative care and hospice care to help a cancer patient through the journey. For example, in their Resources section there are several very useful downloadable "Your Conversation Starter Guide" from The Conversation Project that can help a cancer patient to talk about what matters most through dozens of questions and have a say in their health care. The Guides are divided into 4 steps (think about what matters to you; plan your talk; start talking; keep talking) and emphasizes that "It always seems too soon, until it's too late."

The table below shows the type of care available at Caringinfo with additional information. And the website also has a search tool allowing you to find hospice, palliative care, and bereavement service providers that may be near you.

Service/Resource	Description
Advance Directives	CaringInfo offers free advance directive forms for all 50 states, as well

	as information and guidance on how to complete them.
Hospice Care	CaringInfo provides information and resources on hospice care, including how to choose a hospice provider and what services are typically covered.
Palliative Care	CaringInfo provides information and resources on palliative care, including what it is, how it differs from hospice care, and how to access it.
End-of-Life Care	CaringInfo provides information and resources on end-of-life care, including pain management, symptom control, and emotional support.
Grief Support	CaringInfo offers resources and support for those who are grieving the loss of a loved one, including articles, webinars, and a directory of local grief support services.
Planning for Care	CaringInfo provides guidance on how to plan for long-term care, including information on financing options, legal issues, and caregiver support.
Veterans Care	CaringInfo offers resources for veterans and their families, including information on VA benefits, end-of-life planning, and bereavement support.

Specifically, regarding hospice care, Hospice Foundation of America website (https://hospicefoundation.org) offers a 24-question hospice knowledge quiz that is based on Medicare guidelines and dispels the myths about hospice with detailed answers to each question. A few points to highlight, hospice care tends to be most beneficial when families receive the full range of skilled medical, emotional and spiritual support services for at least a month or more, while grief support is available for the surviving family members up to a year after the patient's death. In many cases, family members provide much of day-to-day patient care; but hospice nurses, social workers and other team members provide education and support to the family caregivers.

ABOUT THE AUTHOR

Dr. Andy Brown

Dr. Andy Brown is an exceptional individual with a profound background in genetics research. Holding a PhD degree in this field, Andy has spent over 10 years to studying the intricacies of genetics and its impact on cancer development, progression, and treatment. His extensive academic training and hands-on experience have equipped him with a deep understanding of the molecular mechanisms underlying various types of cancers.

Beyond his academic achievements, Dr Brown possesses a remarkable passion for spreading knowledge and enhancing patient care. Driven by a genuine desire to make a positive difference in the lives of cancer patients, he has embarked on a mission to bridge the gap between medical expertise and patient understanding. His dedication to empowering patients through education is evident in the meticulous crafting of this practical guide.

Dr. Brown's commitment to providing comprehensive and accessible information stems from his firm belief that informed patients are better equipped to actively participate in their own treatment journey. By distilling complex scientific concepts into easily understandable language, Dr. Brown ensures that readers can grasp the essentials of modern cancer treatments, enabling them to make well-informed decisions and engage in meaningful conversations with their healthcare providers.

www.ingramcontent.com/pod-product-compliance
Lightning Source LLC
Chambersburg PA
CBHW061622250726
48659CB00004B/1050

www.ingramcontent.com/pod-product-compliance
Lightning Source LLC
Chambersburg PA
CBHW050907260726
48660CB00001B/64